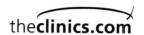

HAND CLINICS

Carpal Disorders

GUEST EDITORS
Steve K. Lee, MD
Michael R. Hausman, MD

November 2006 • Volume 22 • Number 4

SAUNDERS

An Imprint of Elsevier, Inc.
PHILADELPHIA   LONDON   TORONTO   MONTREAL   SYDNEY   TOKYO

W.B. SAUNDERS COMPANY

A Division of Elsevier Inc.

1600 John F. Kennedy Blvd. • Suite 1800 • Philadelphia, Pennsylvania 19103

http://www.theclinics.com

HAND CLINICS   Volume 22, Number 4
November 2006   ISSN 0749-0712
Editor: Debora Dellapena   ISBN 1-4160-3807-8

The ideas and opinions expressed in *Hand Clinics* do not necessarily reflect those of the Publisher. The Publisher does not assume any responsibility for any injury and/or damage to persons or property arising out of or related to any use of the material contained in this periodical. The reader is advised to check the appropriate medical literature and the product information provided by the manufacturer of each drug to be administered to verify the dosage, the method and duration of administration, or contraindications. It is the responsibility of the treating physician or other health care professional, relying on independent experience and knowledge of the patient, to determine drug dosages and the best treatment for the patient. Mention of any product in this issue should not be construed as endorsement by the contributors, editors, or the Publisher of the product or manufacturers' claims.

Hand Clinics (ISSN 0749-0712) is published quarterly by Elsevier Inc., 360 Park Avenue South, New York, NY 10010-1710. Months of publication are February, May, August, and November. Business and Editorial Offices: 1600 John F. Kennedy Blvd., Suite 1800, Philadelphia, PA 19103-2899. Customer Service Office: 6277 Sea Harbor Drive, Orlando, FL 32887-4800. Periodicals postage paid at New York, NY, and additional mailing offices. Subscription price is $237.00 per year (U.S. individuals), $362.00 per year (U.S. institutions), $121.00 per year (US students), $270.00 per year (Canadian individuals), $405.00 per year (Canadian institutions), $149.00 (Canadian students), $303.00 per year (international individuals), $405.00 per year (international institutions), and $149.00 per year (international students). Foreign air speed delivery is included in all *Clinics* subscription prices. All prices are subject to change without notice. POSTMASTER: Send address changes to *Hand Clinics*, Elsevier Periodicals Customer Service, 6277 Sea Harbor Drive, Orlando, FL 32887-4800. **Customer Service: 1-800-654-2452 (US). From outside the US, call 1-407-345-4000. E-mail: hhspcs@harcourt.com.**

Reprints. For copies of 100 or more, of articles in this publication, please contact the Commercial Rights Department, Elsevier Inc., 360 Park Avenue South, New York, NY 10010-1710. Tel: (212) 633-3813, Fax: (212) 462-1935, e-mail: reprints@elsevier.com.

Hand Clinics is covered in *Index Medicus, Current Contents/Clinical Medicine, EMBASE/Excerpta Medica,* and *ISI/BIOMED.*

Printed in the United States of America.

GUEST EDITORS

STEVE K. LEE, MD, Associate Chief, Hand Surgery Service, Department of Orthopaedic Surgery, New York University Hospital for Joint Diseases Orthopaedics Institute; Assistant Professor, The New York University School of Medicine; Co-Chief, Hand Surgery Service, Bellevue Hospital Center; Attending, Department of Orthopedic Surgery, St. Vincent's Hospital Manhattan, New York, New York

MICHAEL R. HAUSMAN, MD, Robert K. Lippman Professor of Orthopaedics; Vice-Chairman, Department of Orthopaedics; Chief, Hand and Elbow Surgery, The Mount Sinai Medical Center, New York, New York

CONTRIBUTORS

ALBERTO AVILES, MD, Fellow, Hand Surgery Service, The Institute of Plastic and Reconstructive Surgery, The New York University School of Medicine, New York, New York

LOUIS CATALANO III, MD, C.V. Starr Hand Surgery Center, Saint Luke's-Roosevelt Hospital, New York, New York

JOSEPH J. CRISCO, PhD, Associate Professor, Department of Orthopaedics, Brown Medical School/Rhode Island Hospital, Providence, Rhode Island

EDWARD DIAO, MD, Chief, Division of Hand, Upper Extremity, and Microvascular Surgery; Professor of Orthopaedic Surgery and Neurosurgery, University of California San Francisco, San Francisco, California

CHRISTOPHER L. FORTHMAN, MD, Attending Hand Surgeon, Curtis National Hand Center, Union Memorial Hospital, Baltimore, Maryland

MICHAEL J. GARDNER, MD, Chief Resident, Department of Orthopaedic Surgery, Hospital for Special Surgery, New York, New York

FRANCESCO GARGANO, MD, Hand Surgery Fellow, Department of Orthopaedic Surgery, The Mount Sinai School of Medicine, New York, New York

RYAN J. GRABOW, MD, Nevada Orthopedic and Spine Center, Las Vegas, Nevada

MICHAEL R. HAUSMAN, MD, Robert K. Lippman Professor of Orthopaedics; Vice-Chairman, Department of Orthopaedics; Chief, Hand and Elbow Surgery, The Mount Sinai Medical Center, New York, New York

PATRICIA A. HSU, MD, Resident, Department of Orthopaedic Surgery and Rehabilitation, Loyola University Chicago Stritch School of Medicine, Maywood, Illinois

ANTHONY J. LAUDER, MD, Fellow in Hand and Microvascular Surgery Program, Department of Orthopaedics and Sports Medicine, University of Washington Medical Center, Seattle, Washington

STEVE K. LEE, MD, Associate Chief, Hand Surgery Service, Department of Orthopaedic Surgery, New York University Hospital for Joint Diseases Orthopaedics Institute; Assistant Professor, The New York University School of Medicine; Co-Chief, Hand Surgery Service, Bellevue Hospital Center; Attending, Department of Orthopedic Surgery, St. Vincent's Hospital Manhattan, New York, New York

TERRY R. LIGHT, MD, The Dr. William M. Scholl Professor and Chairman, Department of Orthopaedic Surgery and Rehabilitation, Loyola University Chicago Stritch School of Medicine, Maywood, Illinois

JEFFREY LUO, MD, Fellow, Hand, Upper Extremity, and Microvascular Surgery, Department of Orthopaedic Surgery, University of California San Francisco, San Francisco, California

MITSUHIKO NANNO, MD, PhD, Division of Hand Surgery, Department of Orthopaedic Surgery, Nippon Medical School, Musashikosugi Hospital, Kawasaki, Japan

RITA M. PATTERSON, PhD, Division of Biomechanics and Bone Physiology Research, Department of Orthopaedic Surgery and Rehabilitation, University of Texas Medical Branch, Galveston, Texas

BRETT PETERSON, MD, Department of Orthopaedic Surgery, University of California Davis School of Medicine, Sacramento, California

KEITH A. SEGALMAN, MD, Assistant Professor, Department of Orthopaedic Surgery, Johns Hopkins School of Medicine, Johns Hopkins University, Baltimore, Maryland

ALEXANDER Y. SHIN, MD, Professor and Consultant, Department of Orthopaedic Surgery, Division of Hand Surgery, Mayo Clinic College of Medicine, Rochester, Minnesota

ROBERT M. SZABO, MD, MPH, Chief, Hand and Upper Extremity Service; Professor of Orthopaedics; Professor of Surgery, Division of Plastic Surgery, University of California Davis School of Medicine, Sacramento, California

SHIAN CHAO TAY, MD, Fellow, Department of Orthopaedic Surgery, Division of Hand Surgery, Mayo Clinic College of Medicine, Rochester, Minnesota; and Associate Consultant, Department of Hand Surgery, Singapore General Hospital, Singapore

THOMAS E. TRUMBLE, MD, Professor and Chief, University of Washington Hand Surgery Institute, Department of Orthopaedics and Sports Medicine, University of Washington Medical Center, Seattle, Washington

STEVEN F. VIEGAS, MD, Professor and Chief, Division of Hand Surgery, Department of Orthopaedic Surgery and Rehabilitation; Professor of Anatomy and Neurosciences; Professor of Preventative Medicine and Community Health, University of Texas Medical Branch, Galveston, Texas

MORDECHAI VIGLER, MD, Fellow, Hand Surgery Service, New York University Hospital for Joint Diseases Orthopaedic Institute, Department of Orthopaedic Surgery, The New York University School of Medicine, New York, New York

SCOTT W. WOLFE, MD, Professor, Department of Orthopaedic Surgery, Hospital for Special Surgery, New York, New York

CONTENTS

for proper management of these serious injuries. In this article the authors address the five main categories of carpal dislocations, the associated anatomy, and their diagnosis, treatment, and prognosis.

Carpal Fractures Excluding the Scaphoid

Mordechai Vigler, Alberto Aviles, and Steve K. Lee

Although carpal fractures other than of the scaphoid are uncommon, vigilance in diagnosing these potentially serious fractures is paramount to early and effective treatment. Physical examination and standard plain radiographs may reveal only subtle findings. Use of special radiographic views and computed tomography may help elucidate the diagnosis. Treatment is particular to each fracture. Nondisplaced fractures should be treated nonoperatively. For intra-articular carpal bone fractures, virtually any amount of displacement is unacceptable and requires reduction and fixation. This article organizes current knowledge of these potentially difficult fractures, with a table of diagnosis and treatment guidelines.

Carpal Osteoarthrosis

Brett Peterson and Robert M. Szabo

Despite improved understanding of carpal mechanics, increased awareness of intercarpal ligament injuries, and improved techniques for treating carpal instability, post-traumatic intercarpal osteoarthrosis remains a common problem. Osteoarthritis of the carpal bones, including scapholunate advance collapse wrist, scaphotrapeziotrapezoid arthritis, lunotriquetral arthritis, triquetrohamate arthritis, and pisotriquetral arthritis, follows specific unique patterns, but in each, the final common pathway leads to degenerative change. Injury or deformity leads to instability and altered kinematics, producing abnormal joint contact pressures. Cartilage injury and eventual degeneration of the joint follow. The etiology, prevalence, and current evaluation and treatment of these conditions are of importance to hand surgeons.

Wrist Arthrofibrosis

Steve K. Lee, Francesco Gargano, and Michael R. Hausman

Wrist arthrofibrosis is a condition of decreased range of wrist motion due to intrinsic adhesions and extrinsic contracture. It is clinically characterized by restricted wrist range of motion, pain, swelling, and a plateau in improvement after at least 6 months of intensive physiotherapy. Other conditions must be excluded, such as articular incongruity, arthritis, spasticity, skin and subcutaneous scarring, and loose bodies. We have devised a classification system based on pathologic anatomic location, where Type I represents intrinsic adhesions, and Type II represents extrinsic contracture. The types are subdivided according to where the pathology is present. The operative approach should be wrist arthroscopy for Types IA (radiocarpal adhesions) and IB (midcarpal adhesions) where intraarticular adhesions are present. Types IC (distal radioulnar joint adhesions) and II C (distal radioulnar joint capsular contracture) are best approached in an open manner where dorsal and palmar capsulectomies of the distal radioulnar joint are performed. For Types IIA, B, and D (dorsal, palmar, and combination extrinsic contracture, respectively), both open and arthroscopic methods are described.

Index

FORTHCOMING ISSUES

RECENT ISSUES

ELSEVIER
SAUNDERS

Hand Clin 22 (2006) ix–x

HAND
CLINICS

Preface

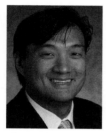 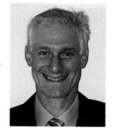

Steve K. Lee, MD   Michael R. Hausman, MD
Guest Editors

Much has been written about the wrist, but in this issue of *Hand Clinics*, we've chosen to highlight topics that have received disproportionately less attention relative to their clinical relevance. In addition, we highlight the work of several authors presenting a new perspective on carpal mechanics. This work was first presented in research publications, but we consider it worthy of wider dissemination, and thus have asked the authors to present their findings in a more discursive format.

To this end, Drs. Wolfe, Gardner, and Crisco discuss their recent analysis of the "dart thrower's motion" that incorporates many disparate thoughts and theories about carpal motion and mechanics. Dr. Viegas's innovative methods and comprehensive analysis complement this study. Transitioning to the operating room, Drs. Shin and Tay summarize the work of the Mayo Clinic on nondestructive surgical approaches to the wrist.

Dr. Light is a recognized authority on congenital hand deformities. For this volume, he and Dr. Tsu focus specifically on congenital disorders of the wrist. We are indebted to Drs. Lauder and Trumble for what is probably the most comprehensive review of Preiser's Disease to date, while Jeffrey Luo and Edward Diao organize the widely divergent theories and treatments of Kienböck's disease.

Tumors and lesions of the carpus have received little specific attention, and Christopher Forthman and Keith Segalman rectify this, while Ryan Grabow and Louis Catalano provide a complete review on dislocations of the carpus. We present carpal fractures other than of the scaphoid and offer new summary tables that should help as quick reference guides.

Alleviating pain associated with osteoarthrosis of the carpus while preserving motion remains a frequent challenge and Drs. Peterson and Szabo review current therapies and share their strategies for treating this condition. Finally, apropos of motion, we address the issue of arthrofibrosis of the wrist; a diagnosis that is usually treatable, but is infrequently entertained for posttraumatic motion lost at the wrist.

It has been an honor and privilege to serve as Guest Editors for this edition of *Hand Clinics*. We are indebted to our authors and to editors

doi:10.1016/j.hcl.2006.09.001

Deb Dellapena and Patrick Manley for their encouragement and assistance.

Steve K. Lee, MD
New York University Hospital for Joint Diseases
Orthopaedics Institute
The New York University School of Medicine
301 East 17th Street
New York, NY 10003, USA

E-mail address: steve.lee@nyumc.org

Michael R. Hausman, MD
Department of Orthopaedic Surgery
The Mount Sinai Medical Center
5 East 98th Street, Box 1188
New York, NY 10029, USA

E-mail address:
michael.hausman@msnyuhealth.org

HAND
CLINICS

Hand Clin 22 (2006) 399–412

Three-Dimensional Imaging of the Carpal Ligaments

Mitsuhiko Nanno, MD, PhD[a], Rita M. Patterson, PhD[b],
Steven F. Viegas, MD[b],*

[a]*Division of Hand Surgery, Department of Orthopaedic Surgery, Nippon Medical School,
Musashikosugi Hospital 1-396, Kosugicho, Nakahara-ku, Kawasaki 211-8533, Japan*
[b]*Department of Orthopaedic Surgery and Rehabilitation, University of Texas Medical Branch,
301 University Boulevard, Galveston, TX 77555-0165, USA*

Although many articles have examined the anatomy and function of the carpal ligaments [1–20], these remain incompletely understood. Visualization all of the ligaments of the wrist during surgery is almost impossible. Many carpal and metacarpal ligaments cannot be seen unless the extrinsic ligaments and tendons are incised or removed. Recent studies describe the anatomic and mechanical properties of the carpometacarpal (CMC) ligaments [1,2], but little three-dimensional (3-D) information is available detailing the specific location and area of ligament attachments on the individual carpal and metacarpal bones [3]. Successful diagnosis of injuries, interpretation of images, and treatment depend on accurate knowledge of the anatomic ligament attachment locations [3].

This article provides a new perspective and detailed anatomic description of the attachments of the CMC ligaments, intercarpal ligaments, and radiocarpal ligaments, which are described and illustrated using a unique combination of detailed dissection, CT imaging, and 3-D digitization. The discussion ties together previously published descriptions [3] and the most recent insights into the anatomy of the wrist ligaments. Detailed information is also provided about the ligamentous attachments of the CMC joints, carpal bones, and distal radius. This information advances the current knowledge and understanding of the normal anatomy and its impact on the mechanics of the radiocarpal intercarpal ligaments and the CMC joints, and should help surgeons to assess and treat injuries and degenerative changes seen in the wrist and CMC joints.

The carpometacarpal ligaments and the intermetacarpal ligaments

Many investigators have studied the anatomy of the first CMC joint ligaments [1,4–13]. Weitbrecht [4] reported that the first CMC joint contained three ligaments: palmar, dorsal, and lateral. Haines [5], Napier [6], von Lanz and Wachsmuth [7], Spinner [8], Pieron [9], Pagalidis and colleagues [10], Drewniany and colleagues [11], Pellegrini [12], and Imaeda and colleagues [13] further detailed this anatomy. Most recently, Bettinger and colleagues [1] described the complex ligamentous anatomy of the trapezium and trapeziometacarpal joint, and identified the superficial anterior oblique ligament (SAOL), deep anterior oblique ligament (dAOL), ulnar collateral ligament (UCL), dorsoradial ligament (DRL), and posterior oblique ligament (POL) of the first CMC joint. They also described the volar intermetacarpal ligament, dorsal intermetacarpal ligament in the intermetacarpal joint, dorsal trapezium–trapezoid ligament, volar trapezium–trapezoid ligament, dorsal trapezium–second metacarpal ligament, volar trapezium–second metacarpal ligament, volar trapezium–third metacarpal ligament, transverse carpal ligament, and trapezoid–capitate ligament [1]. Although the first CMC joint is a common area of surgical exposure and treatment, the anatomy of the ligaments remains incompletely understood and is typically not visualized.

* Corresponding author.
E-mail address: sviegas@utmb.edu (S.F. Viegas).

0749-0712/06/$ - see front matter © 2006 Elsevier Inc. All rights reserved.
doi:10.1016/j.hcl.2006.08.003

Table 1
Individual ligament attachments of the volar, dorsal, and interosseous ligaments on the metacarpals and carpal bones in the carpometacarpal and intermetacarpal joints

Ligaments	Location	Area (mm^2)	Specimens (N = 6)
The carpometacarpal ligaments			
Dorsal ligaments			
DRL			6
	1MC	14.6 ± 3.0	
	Tm	21.5 ± 7.8	
POL			6
	1MC	28.0 ± 9.0	
	Tm	26.9 ± 2.7	
d 2MC rb–Tm ligament			6
	2MC	8.7 ± 2.7	
	Tm	16.8 ± 7.8	
d 2MC rb–Td ligament			6
	2MC	11.3 ± 7.7	
	Td	11.7 ± 4.4	
d 2MC ub–Td ligament			6
	2MC	11.6 ± 4.8	
	Td	8.7 ± 3.8	
d 3MC rb–Td ligament			6
	3MC	6.0 ± 2.7	
	Td	7.3 ± 2.6	
d 3MC rb–C ligament			6
	3MC	11.1 ± 4.7	
	C	7.8 ± 3.1	
d 3MC ub–C–H–4MC rb ligament			2
	3MC	13.4 ± 3.5	
	4MC	7.9 ± 1.2	
	C	5.8 ± 2.2	
	H	2.7 ± 0.5	
d 3MC ub–C–4MC rb ligament			4
	3MC	17.2 ± 1.9	
	4MC	6.6 ± 2.0	
	C	8.5 ± 2.3	
d 4MC ub–H ligament			5
	4MC	11.3 ± 4.4	
	H	8.0 ± 3.1	
d 4MC ub–H–5MC ligament			5
	4MC	4.9 ± 1.8	
	H	8.9 ± 5.0	
	5MC	8.0 ± 3.8	
d 5MC ub–H ligament			6
	5MC	8.4 ± 4.2	
	H	9.0 ± 3.9	
Volar ligaments			
SAOL			6
	1MC	25.8 ± 5.9	
	Tm	36.8 ± 7.4	
dSOL			5
	1MC	9.8 ± 3.5	
	Tm	9.6 ± 5.0	
UCL			6
	1MC	9.5 ± 2.9	
v 2MC rb–Tm ligament			6
	2MC	8.1 ± 4.9	

(continued on next page)

Table 1 (*continued*)

Ligaments	Location	Area (mm^2)	Specimens (N = 6)
	Tm	7.2 ± 2.8	
v 2MC–Td ligament			6
	2MC	7.7 ± 3.4	
	Td	10.5 ± 5.8	
v 3MC rb–Tm ligament			6
	3MC	4.6 ± 1.5	
	Tm	5.1 ± 0.4	
v 3MC–C ligament			6
	3MC	7.2 ± 3.5	
	C	7.1 ± 1.9	
v 3MC–H ligament			5
	3MC	5.1 ± 2.2	
	H	3.2 ± 0.6	
v 4MC–H ligament			3
	4MC	4.9 ± 1.4	
	H	7.9 ± 1.8	
v 4MC–HH ligament			3
	4MC	3.3 ± 1.1	
	H	6.2 ± 1.1	
v 5MC–HH ligament			6
	5MC	11.2 ± 3.0	
	HH	14.9 ± 6.1	
v 5MC–H ligament			1
	5MC	4.3	
	H	6.5	
Interosseous ligament			
2MC–Tm interosseous ligament			6
	2nd MC	13.9 ± 6.2	
	Tm	12.4 ± 6.5	
Intermetacarpal ligament			
Dorsal ligaments			
d 1MC ub–2MC rb intermetacarpal ligament			6
	1MC	12.2 ± 4.2	
	2MC	16.2 ± 4.2	
d 2MC ub dist–3MC rb dist intermetacarpal ligament			4
	2MC	5.8 ± 4.4	
	3MC	12.0 ± 5.3	
d 2MC ub prox–3MC rb prox intermetacarpal ligament			6
	2MC	14.1 ± 8.5	
	3MC	14.8 ± 11.3	
d 3MC ub–4MC rb intermetacarpal ligament			6
	3MC	10.7 ± 2.9	
	4MC	8.5 ± 3.0	
d 4MC ub–5MC rb intermetacarpal ligament			6
	4MC	11.3 ± 4.9	
	5MC	11.2 ± 6.7	
volar ligaments			
v 1MC ub–2MC rb intermetacarpal ligament			6
	1MC	9.7 ± 2.3	

(*continued on next page*)

Table 1 (*continued*)

Ligaments	Location	Area (mm^2)	Specimens (N = 6)
	2MC	11.0 ± 3.0	
v 2MC ub–3MC rb intermetacarpal ligament			6
	2MC	13.9 ± 5.1	
	3MC	13.5 ± 6.4	
v 3MC ub–4MC rb intermetacarpal ligament			6
	3MC	14.5 ± 4.4	
	4MC	15.0 ± 8.0	
v 4MC ub–5MC rb intermetacarpal ligament			6
	4MC	18.7 ± 6.9	
	5MC	15.8 ± 6.1	
v 3MC–4MC–5MC intermetacarpal ligament			6
	3MC	15.6 ± 8.9	
	4MC	7.15 ± 2.6	
	5MC	12.4 ± 7.4	
Interosseous ligament			
2MC–3MC intermetacarpal interosseous ligament			6
	2MC	19.8 ± 16.3	
	3MC	20.9 ± 12.3	
3MC–4MC intermetacarpal interosseous ligament			6
	3MC	14.2 ± 4.9	
	4MC	10.9 ± 4.5	
4MC–5MC intermetacarpal interosseous ligament			6
	4MC	12.2 ± 2.3	
	5MC	10.8 ± 6.2	
Intra–articular ligament			
3rd/4th MC–C/H intra–articular ligament			6
	3MC	20.2 ± 7.3	
	4MC	13.5 ± 3.5	
	C	19.0 ± 5.6	
	H	19.3 ± 4.9	
The intercarpal ligaments			
Dorsal ligaments			
d Tm–Td ligament			6
	Tm	27.1 ± 12.9	
	Td	12.4 ± 5.5	
d Td–C ligament			6
	Td	9.2 ± 2.5	
	C	8.3 ± 4.0	
d C dist–H dist ligament			6
	C	10.1 ± 4.7	
	H	8.6 ± 4.5	
d C prox–H prox ligament			6
	C	7.1 ± 2.9+	
	H	8.0 ± 2.7	
Volar ligaments			
v Tm–Td ligament			6

(*continued on next page*)

Table 1 (*continued*)

Ligaments	Location	Area (mm^2)	Specimens (N = 6)
	Tm	10.6 ± 5.1	
	Td	11.8 ± 5.0	
v Tm–S rb ligament			6
	Tm	11.3 ± 6.7	
	S	8.0 ± 1.5	
v Tm–S ub ligament			5
	Tm	8.8 ± 3.5	
	S	7.5 ± 2.3	
v Tm–C ligament			6
	Tm	14.0 ± 9.3	
	C	9.4 ± 3.0	
v Td–S ligament			6
	Td	4.8 ± 2.0	
	S	4.8 ± 1.2	
v Td–C ligament			6
	Td	10.4 ± 5.3	
	C	12.3 ± 6.5	
v S–C ligament			6
	S	66.7 ± 6.1	
	C	11.7 ± 5.2	
v C–H ligament			6
	C	21.0 ± 8.9	
	H	22.2 ± 8.4	
Interosseous ligaments			
Tm–Td interosseous ligament			6
	Tm	4.5 ± 1.2	
	Td	6.2 ± 2.1	
Td–C interosseous ligament			6
	Td	13.0 ± 5.6	
	C	17.5 ± 5.7	
C–H interosseous ligament			6
	C	26.1 ± 8.7	
	H	22.1 ± 4.9	

Abbreviations: C, capitate; d, dorsal; dist, distal; DRL, dorsoradial ligament; dSOL, deep anterior oblique ligament; H, hamate; HH, hook of the hamate; MC, metacarpal; POL, posterior oblique ligament; prox, proximal; rb, radial base; S, scaphoid; SAOL, superficial anterior oblique ligament; Td, trapezoid; Tm, trapezium; ub, ulnar base; UCL, ulnar collateral ligament; v, volar.

In contrast, the descriptions of the ligamental and skeletal anatomy of the second through fifth CMC joints are neither as detailed nor as extensively reported. Harwin and colleagues [14] described the dorsal ligaments of the bases of the second through fifth metacarpal. Although the second through fourth metacarpals had two dorsal ligaments each, the fifth metacarpal had only one dorsal ligament. They described a similar configuration for the palmar ligaments, except that the third metacarpal had three ligaments attached [14]. Joseph and colleagues [15] reported that the second metacarpal had three dorsal and three volar ligaments, whereas the third metacarpal had two dorsal and three volar ligaments and the fourth

had two dorsal ligaments. Gurland [16] later stated that collectively the CMC joints had six volar and six dorsal ligaments that held them together.

More recently, Nakamura and colleagues [2] published a detailed study of the ligament and skeletal anatomy of these joints and their adjacent structures. They found that the second, third, fourth, and fifth metacarpals each had two dorsal CMC ligaments, and that the second, fourth, and fifth metacarpals each had one volar CMC ligament, whereas the third metacarpal had four distinct volar CMC ligaments [2]. They also reported that many dorsal and volar intermetacarpal ligaments connected the bases of the second through fifth metacarpals, and cited only one

Table 2

Individual ligament attachments of the volar, dorsal, and interosseous ligaments on the metacarpals and carpal bones in radiocarpal and intercarpal joints

Ligaments	Location	Area (mm²)	Specimens (N = 8)
The radiocarpal and intercarpal ligaments			
Dorsal ligaments			
DRC			
	Radius	14.3 ± 4.0	8
	Lunate	1.9 ± 0.6	4
	Triquetrum	8.5 ± 5.4	8
DIC			
	Triquetrum	9.7 ± 6.4	8
	Lunate	3.8 ± 1.3	6
	Scaphoid		
	Proximal	5.7 ± 2.3	8
	Waist	5.2 ± 3.2	6
	Trapezoid	4.0 ± 2.3	8
	Trapezium	2.4	1
Volar ligaments			
LRL			
	Radius	10.9 ± 2.9	8
	Lunate	7.6 ± 2.5	8
SRL			5
	Radius	12.8 ± 3.8	8
	Lunate	13.7 ± 5.6	8
RSL			6
	Radius	5.0 ± 1.7	8
	Scaphoid	3.2 ± 1.9	8
	Lunate	5.5 ± 3.2	8
UL			
	Lunate	2.7 ± 2.7	4
LT			
	Lunate	3.8 ± 2.2	7
	Triquetrum	2.8 ± 0.8	7
Interosseous ligaments			
SLIO			
	Volar		
	Scaphoid	4.7 ± 1.7	8
	Lunate	4.9 ± 1.8	8
	Proximal		
	Scaphoid	13.7 ± 7.0	8
	Lunate	16.3 ± 5.6	8
	Dorsal		
	Scaphoid	4.9 ± 0.8	8
	Lunate	4.9 ± 2.4	8
LTIO			
	Volar		
	Lunate	5.8 ± 2.1	8
	Triquetrum	5.2 ± 2.2	8
	Proximal		
	Lunate	14.4 ± 4.6	8
	Triquetrum	11.7 ± 3.7	8
	Dorsal		
	Lunate	3.9 ± 2.8	8
	Triquetrum	2.2 ± 0.9	8

Abbreviations: DIC, dorsal intercarpal; DRC, dorsal radiocarpal; LRI, long radiolunate ligament; LT, lunotriquetral; LTIO, lunotriquetral interosseous; SLIO, scapholunate interosseous; SRL, short radiolunate ligament; RSL, radioscapholunate; UL, ulnolunate.

From Nagao S, Patterson RM, Buford WL, et al. Three-dimensional description of ligamentous attachments around the lunate. J Hand Surg [Am] 2005;30:687; with permission from The American Society for Surgery of the Hand.

intra-articular ligament located between the third and fourth metacarpals and the capitate and the hamate. This ligament provided stability even when the dorsal and volar CMC ligaments were cut, but was not found in 4% of the specimens. The specimens without the intra-articular ligament had a single narrow articulation between the fourth metacarpal and the hamate, which was the type III anatomy described by Viegas and colleagues [21].

A more detailed ligament anatomy

Using 3-D digitization and CT reconstructions with careful dissection, researchers were recently able visualize and quantify the anatomy and specific area and locations of ligament attachments on the individual carpal bones, metacarpals, and distal radius. Nagao and colleagues [3] and Nanno and colleagues [22,23] took CT images of the hands they researched and then recreated the bone structure in a 3-D image. They also rendered the ligament attachment sites and areas in 3-D. The images of the bone structures and ligaments were then combined to provide a complete picture. These studies described the ligament attachment areas in square millimeters (mean ± SD) (Tables 1 and 2) and noted the presence or absence of each ligament.

Dorsal carpometacarpal ligaments

Nanno and colleagues [22,23] found and identified multiple dorsal CMC ligaments, including two dorsal ligaments that attached to the first metacarpal, extending from the dorsoradial or dorsal base of the first metacarpal to the trapezium (DRL and POL). They also identified three distinct dorsal ligaments attached to the second metacarpal [18]. One extended from the radial base of the second metacarpal to the trapezoid (d 2MC rb–Td), whereas the second extended from the ulnar base of the second metacarpal to the trapezoid (d 2MC ub–Td). The third extended from the radial base of the second metacarpal to the trapezium (d 2MC rb–Tm) (Fig. 1).

They also identified three distinct dorsal ligaments that attached to the third metacarpal base. One extended from the radial base of the third metacarpal to the trapezoid (d 3MC rb–Td) (Fig. 2). The second extended from the radial base of the third metacarpal to the capitate (d 3MC rb–C). The third extended from the ulnar base of the third metacarpal to the capitate and

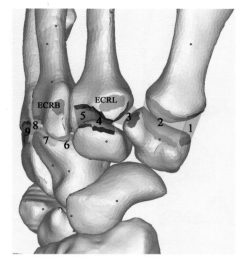

Fig. 1. A dorsoradial view of a 3-D model of a left wrist. The solid, colored areas show ligament attachment and the transparent colored areas show the paths of the ligaments. (*1*) Dorsoradial ligament. (*2*) Posterior oblique ligament. (*3*) Dorsal second metacarpal radial base–trapezium ligament. (*4*) Dorsal second metacarpal radial base–trapezoid ligament. (*5*) Dorsal second metacarpal ulnar base–trapezoid ligament. (*6*) Dorsal third metacarpal radial base–trapezoid ligament. (*7*) Dorsal third metacarpal radial base–capitate ligament. (*8*) Dorsal third metacarpal ulnar base–capitate–hamate fourth metacarpal radial base ligament. (*9*) Dorsal fourth metacarpal ulnar base–hamate ligament. ECRB, extensor carpi radialis brevis; ECRL, extensor carpi radialis longus.

to the radial base of the fourth metacarpal (d 3MC ub–C–4MC rb) and, in some cases, also extended to the hamate (d 3MC ub–C–H–4MC rb).

Nanno and colleagues [23] also identified three distinct dorsal ligaments that attached to the fourth metacarpal base. The first extended from the dorsal base of the fourth metacarpal to the hamate (d 4MC ub–H). The second extended from the radial base of the fourth metacarpal to the capitate and the ulnar base of the third metacarpal (d 3MC ub–C–4MC rb) and, in some cases, also extended to the hamate (d 3MC ub–C–H–4MC rb). The third extended from the ulnar base of the fourth metacarpal to the hamate and the radial base of the fifth metacarpal (d 4MC ub–H–5MC rb). They also identified two distinct dorsal ligaments attached to the dorsal aspect of the fifth metacarpal. One extended from the ulnar base of the fifth metacarpal to the hamate (d 5MC ub–H), whereas the second extended from the radial base

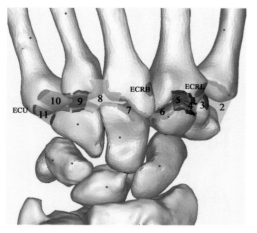

Fig. 2. A dorsal view of a 3-D model of a left wrist. The solid, colored areas show ligament attachment and the transparent colored areas show the paths of the ligaments. (2) Posterior oblique ligament. (3) Dorsal second metacarpal radial base–trapezium ligament. (4) Dorsal second metacarpal radial base–trapezoid ligament. (5) Dorsal second metacarpal ulnar base–trapezoid ligament. (6) Dorsal third metacarpal radial base–trapezoid ligament. (7) Dorsal third metacarpal radial base–capitate ligament. (8) Dorsal third metacarpal ulnar base–capitate–hamate fourth metacarpal radial base ligament. (9) Dorsal fourth metacarpal ulnar base–hamate ligament. (10) Dorsal fourth metacarpal ulnar base–hamate–fifth metacarpal radial base ligament. (11) Dorsal fifth metacarpal ulnar base–hamate ligament. ECRB, extensor carpi radialis brevis; ECRL, extensor carpi radialis longus; ECU, extensor carpi ulnaris.

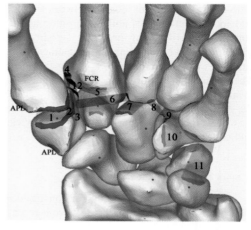

Fig. 3. A volarulnar view of a 3-D model of a left wrist. The solid, colored areas show ligament attachment and the transparent colored areas show the paths of the ligaments. (1) Superficial anterior oblique ligament. (2) Deep anterior oblique ligament. (3) Ulnar collateral ligament. (4) Volar second metacarpal–trapezium ligament. (5) Volar second metacarpal–trapezoid ligament. (6) Volar third metacarpal radial base–trapezium ligament. (7) Volar third metacarpal–capitate ligament. (8) Volar third metacarpal ulnar base–hamate ligament. (9) Volar fourth metacarpal ulnar base–hook of hamate ligament. (10) Volar fifth metacarpal–hook of hamate ligament. (11) Volar fifth metacarpal–pisiform ligament. (12) Second metacarpal–trapezium interosseous ligament. APL, abductor pollicis longus; FCR, flexor carpi radialis.

of the fifth metacarpal to the hamate and the ulnar base of the fourth metacarpal (d 4MC ub–H–5MC rb).

Volar carpometacarpal ligaments

Nanno and colleagues [22,23] also identified multiple volar ligaments, including three distinct volar ligaments that attached to the first metacarpal. The first extended from the volar base of the first metacarpal to the trapezium (SAOL), whereas the second extended from the ulnar base of the first metacarpal to the trapezium (dAOL) (Fig. 3). The third extended from the ulnar base of the first metacarpal to the transverse carpal ligament (UCL). They also identified two distinct volar ligaments that attached to the second metacarpal. One extended from the radial base of the second metacarpal to the trapezium (v 2MC–Tm) and the other extended from the volar base of the second metacarpal to the trapezoid (v 2MC–Td).

These investigators also identified three distinct volar ligaments attached to the third metacarpal [23]. The first extended from the radial base of the third metacarpal to the trapezium (v 3MC rb–Tm) (Fig. 4), the second extended from the volar base of the third metacarpal to the capitate (v 3MC–C), and the third extended from the ulnar base of the third metacarpal to the hamate (v 3MC ub–H). They also identified two distinct volar ligaments that attached to the fourth metacarpal. One extended from the radial base of the fourth metacarpal to the hamate (v 4MC rb–H) and the other extended from the volar base of the fourth metacarpal to the hook of the hamate (v 4MC ub–HH). Furthermore, they identified three distinct volar ligaments that attached to the fifth metacarpal. The first extended from the volar base of the fifth metacarpal to the hook of the hamate (v 5MC–HH), the second extended from the ulnar base of the fifth metacarpal to the hamate (v 5MC–H), and the third extended from the ulnar base of the fifth metacarpal to the pisiform (v 5MC–P).

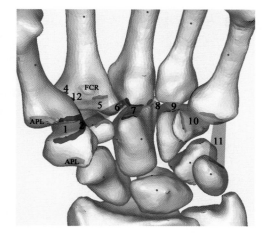

Fig. 4. A volar view of a 3-D model of a left wrist. The solid, colored areas show ligament attachment and the transparent colored areas show the paths of the ligaments. (*1*) Superficial anterior oblique ligament. (*2*) Deep anterior oblique ligament. (*4*) Volar second metacarpal–trapezium ligament. (*5*) Volar second metacarpal–trapezoid ligament. (*6*) Volar third metacarpal radial base–trapezium ligament. (*7*) Volar third metacarpal–capitate ligament. (*8*) Volar third metacarpal ulnar base–hamate ligament. (*9*) Volar fourth metacarpal ulnar base–hook of hamate ligament. (*10*) Volar fifth metacarpal-hook of hamate ligament. (*11*) Volar fifth metacarpal–pisiform ligament. (*12*) Second metacarpal–trapezium interosseous ligament. APL, abductor pollicis longus; FCR, flexor carpi radialis.

These authors located one CMC interosseous ligament that connected the second metacarpal to the trapezium (2MC–Tm IO) (Fig. 3). They located only one intra-articular ligament, which was found between the third metacarpal, fourth metacarpal, capitate, and hamate (3MC/4MC–C/H) (Fig. 5A–C).

Intermetacarpal ligaments

Nanno and colleagues [22,23] identified five dorsal intermetacarpal ligaments: (1) the dorsal first metacarpal ulnar base–second metacarpal radial base (d 1MC ub–2MC rb), (2) the dorsal second metacarpal ulnar base distal–third metacarpal radial base distal (d 2MC ub dist–3MC rb dist), (3) the dorsal second metacarpal ulnar base proximal–third metacarpal radial base proximal (d 2MC ub prox–3MC rb prox), (4) the dorsal third metacarpal ulnar base–fourth metacarpal radial base (d 3MC ub–4MC rb), and (5) the dorsal fourth metacarpal ulnar base–fifth

metacarpal radial base (d 4MC ub–5MC rb) (Fig. 6).

These authors also identified five volar intermetacarpal ligaments: (1) the volar first metacarpal ulnar base–second metacarpal radial base (v 1MC ub–2MC rb), (2) the volar second metacarpal ulnar base–third metacarpal radial base (v 2MC ub dist–3MC rb), (3) the volar third metacarpal ulnar base–fourth metacarpal radial base (v 3MC ub–4MC rb), (4) the volar fourth metacarpal ulnar base–fifth metacarpal radial base (v 4MC ub–5MC rb), and (5) the volar third metacarpal–fourth metacarpal–fifth metacarpal ligament (v 3MC–4MC–5MC) (Fig. 7) [22,23].

They also identified three intermetacarpal interosseous ligaments: (1) the second metacarpal ulnar base–third metacarpal radial base interosseous ligament (2MC ub dist–3MC rb IO), (2) the third metacarpal ulnar base–fourth metacarpal radial base interosseous ligament (3MC ub–4MC rb IO), and (3) the fourth metacarpal ulnar base–fifth metacarpal radial base interosseous ligament (4MC ub–5MC rb IO) (Fig. 7).

The first CMC joint ligament anatomy these authors identified [22] concurred with the previous descriptions by Bettinger and colleagues [1]. Nanno and colleagues found CMC ligaments (SAOL, dAOL, and UCL) that had substantial attachments to the ulnovolar side of the first metacarpal. These strong ligament attachments to the ulnovolar base of the first metacarpal may explain the fracture pattern in a Bennett's fracture dislocation. The volar base of the first metacarpal most likely remains reduced because of these ligament attachments. The remaining first metacarpal, which fractures free from this fragment, dislocates with the pull of the abductor pollicis longus. Furthermore, the radial base of the first metacarpal had a relative paucity of ligaments stabilizing that portion of the thumb CMC joint. The DRL, although thicker than the SAOL, dAOL, and UCL, was the only ligament attached on the posteroradial side of the first metacarpal.

In studying the pathomechanics and pathoanatomy of fracture dislocations of the ring and small finger CMC joints, Yoshida and colleagues [24] found a correlation between fracture sites and the ligament attachment locations described by Nakamura and colleagues [2]. Nakamura and colleagues previously described nine dorsal ligaments and seven volar ligaments of the second through fifth CMC joints. Comparatively, Nanno and colleagues [23] identified 11 dorsal ligaments and 10

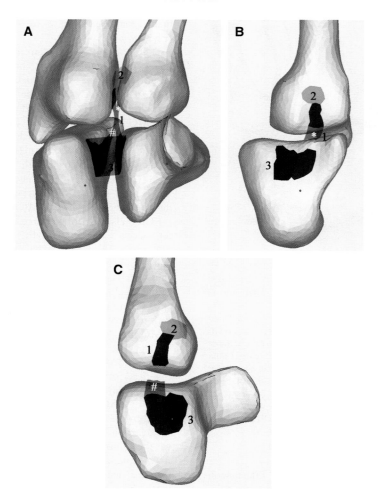

Fig. 5. (*A*) An open-book volar view of the right third metacarpal–fourth metacarpal and capitate–hamate joint. This model is the equivalent of opening the third metacarpal–fourth metacarpal joint and the capitate–hamate joint from the volar side, and was made from individual digitized models by means of computer manipulation. (*B*) The capitate–third metacarpal can be viewed from the ulnar side. (*C*) The hamate–fourth metacarpal can be viewed from the radial side. The solid, colored areas show ligament attachment and the transparent colored areas show the paths of the ligaments. (*1*) Third/fourth metacarpal–capitate/hamate intra–articular ligament. (*2*) Third metacarpal ulnar base–fourth metacarpal radial base interosseous ligament. (*3*) Capitate–hamate interosseous ligament. The portion of ligament connected to the fourth metacarpal (*) and the portion of ligament connected to the capitate (#) are also indicated.

volar ligaments, which include a previously undescribed volar third, fourth, and fifth metacarpal ligament (3MC–4MC–5MC). The volar 3MC–4MC–5MC ligament attached at the volar aspect of the third through fifth metacarpal bases in all six specimens in their study. This ligament was located more volar than the intermetacarpal ligaments.

The location of the ligaments around the second CMC joint by way of the trapezoid to the trapezium is complicated. The UCL, flexor carpi radialis, v 3MC rb–Tm ligament, and v 2MC–Td ligament were situated in turn from top to bottom. Some variation occurred in the second through the fifth CMC ligaments in the study by Nanno and colleagues [23]. They found two variations of the d 3MC ub–C–4MC rb ligament and the d 3MC ub–C–H–4MC rb ligament in the dorsal third and fourth CMC joint. Each ligament existed whether or not the fourth metacarpal articulated with the capitate. The d 4MC ub–H–5MC rb ligament was found on the dorsal side

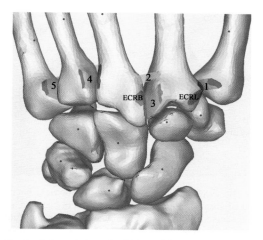

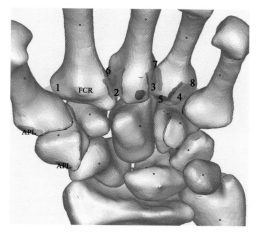

Fig. 6. A dorsal view of a 3-D model of a left wrist. The solid, colored areas show ligament attachment and the transparent colored areas show the paths of the ligaments. (*1*) Dorsal first metacarpal ulnar base–second metacarpal radial base ligament. (*2*) Dorsal second metacarpal ulnar base distal–third metacarpal radial base distal ligament. (*3*) Dorsal second metacarpal ulnar base proximal–third metacarpal radial base proximal ligament. (*4*) Dorsal third metacarpal ulnar base–fourth metacarpal radial base ligament. (*5*) Dorsal fourth metacarpal ulnar base–fifth metacarpal radial base ligament. ECRB, extensor carpi radialis brevis; ECRL, extensor carpi radialis longus.

Fig. 7. A volar distal view of a 3-D model of a left wrist. The solid, colored areas show ligament attachment and the transparent colored areas show the paths of the ligaments. (*1*) Volar first metacarpal ulnar base–second metacarpal radial base ligament. (*2*) Volar second metacarpal ulnar base–third metacarpal radial base ligament. (*3*) Volar third metacarpal ulnar base–fourth metacarpal radial base ligament. (*4*) Volar fourth metacarpal ulnar base–fifth metacarpal radial base ligament. (*5*) Volar third metacarpal–fourth metacarpal–fifth metacarpal ligament. (*6*) Second metacarpal ulnar base–third metacarpal radial base interosseous ligament. (*7*) Third metacarpal ulnar base–fourth metacarpal radial base interosseous ligament. (*8*) Fourth metacarpal ulnar base–fifth metacarpal radial base interosseous ligament. APL, abductor pollicis longus; FCR, flexor carpi radialis.

of the fourth and fifth metacarpal joint. This finding could explain the high incidence of hamate fracture fragments in fourth and fifth CMC joint fracture-dislocations resulting from fist blow injuries, as described by Yoshida and colleagues [24].

Radiocarpal and intercarpal ligaments

Several authors have reported their findings on the radiocarpal and intercarpal ligaments. Berger [17,18] reported the anatomy of the ligaments of the radiocarpal joint and the intercarpal joints of the proximal carpal row, including the long radiolunate ligament, short radiolunate ligament, radioscapholunate ligament, scapholunate interosseous ligament (SLIO), lunotriquetral interosseous ligament (LTIO), dorsal radiocarpal ligament, and dorsal intercarpal ligament.

Nagao and colleagues [3] recently detailed the anatomy of these ligaments, providing more information about the anatomy of the lunotriquetral ligament and the ulnolunate in eight specimens (Table 2). They identified two dorsal ligaments of the lunate and adjacent carpal bones (DRC

and dorsal intercarpal ligaments), reporting that these dorsal ligaments occupied approximately 15% of all ligament attachments on the lunate. They found that the dorsal intercarpal ligament routinely attached to the dorsal aspect of the lunate and the scaphoid and triquetrum. They described the location and area of specific ligamentous attachments on the 3-D surface morphology of the individual carpal bones and distal radius (Figs. 8 and 9) [3]. They also identified five volar ligaments of the lunate and adjacent carpal bones (the long radiolunate, short radiolunate, radioscapholunate, ulnolunate, and lunotriquetral ligaments), reporting that these ligaments composed approximately 49% of all ligament attachments on the lunate (Fig. 10). Moreover, they identified two interosseous ligaments of the lunate and adjacent carpal bones (SLIO and LTIO). The SLIO and LTIO were described as having three parts: a volar portion (vSLIO and vLTIO,

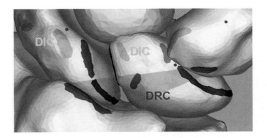

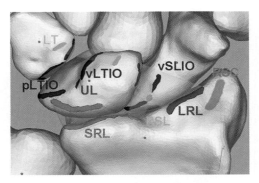

Fig. 8. A dorsal view of the 3-D models of a right wrist joint. Colored areas show ligament attachment and transparent colored areas show the path of the ligaments. DIC, dorsal intercarpal ligament; DRC, dorsal radio-carpal ligament. (*From* Nagao S, Patterson RM, Buford WL, et al. Three-dimensional description of ligamentous attachments around the lunate. J Hand Surg [Am] 2005;30:690; with permission from The American Society for Surgery of the Hand.)

Fig. 10. A volar view of 3-D models of the right lunate and adjacent carpal bones with the areas of ligament attachments identified by different colors. The transparent areas show the path of the ligaments. LRL, long radiolunate ligament; LT, lunotriquetral ligament; pLTIO, proximal portion of the lunotriquetral interosseous ligament; RSC, radioscaphocapitate ligament; RSL, radioscapholunate ligament; SRL, short radiolunate ligament; UL, ulnolunate ligament; vLTIO, volar portion of lunotriquetral interosseous ligament; vSLIO, volar portion of the scapholunate interosseous ligament. (*From* Nagao S, Patterson RM, Buford WL, et al. Three-dimensional description of ligamentous attachments around the lunate. J Hand Surg [Am] 2005;30:689; with permission from The American Society for Surgery of the Hand.)

respectively), a proximal (membranous) portion (pSLIO and pLTIO, respectively), and a dorsal portion (dSLIO and dLTIO, respectively).

Nanno and colleagues [22,23] also recently studied the ligamentous attachments of the distal carpal row. They identified the dorsal trapezium–trapezoid (d Tm–Td) ligament, dorsal trapezoid–capitate (d Td–C) ligament, dorsal capitate–hamate distal (d C–H distal) ligament, and dorsal capitate–hamate proximal (d C–H prox) ligament (Fig. 11). They also identified the

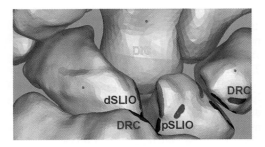

Fig. 9. A dorsal view of the 3-D models of a right wrist joint. Colored areas indicate ligament attachment and transparent colored areas show the path of the ligaments. DIC, dorsal intercarpal ligament. DRC, dorsal radiocarpal ligament; dSLIO, dorsal portion of the scapholunate interosseous ligament; pSLIO, proximal portion of the scapholunate interosseous ligament. (*From* Nagao S, Patterson RM, Buford WL, et al. Three-dimensional description of ligamentous attachments around the lunate. J Hand Surg [Am] 2005;30:691; with permission from The American Society for Surgery of the Hand.)

volar trapezium–trapezoid (v Tm–Td) ligament, volar trapezium–capitate (v Tm–C) ligament, volar trapezoid–capitate (v Td–C) ligament, volar capitate–hamate (v C–H) ligament, trapezium–trapezoid interosseous (Tm–Td IO) ligament (Fig. 12), trapezoid–capitate interosseous (Td–C IO) ligament (Fig. 11), and capite–hamate interosseous (C–H IO) ligament (Fig. 5A).

Nagao and colleagues [3] reported that the ligament anatomy they identified coincided with what Berger [17] described, with the exception of the ulnolunate, LTIO, and dorsal intercarpal ligaments. Berger stated that the ulnolunate ligament was adjacent to the short radiolunate ligament, whereas Nagao and colleagues stated that the ulnolunate ligament was not located at the same level as the short radiolunate ligament, but that it ran parallel to the ulnocapitate and ulnotriquetral ligaments and originated just radial to their attachments at the base of the ulnar styloid process [3]. Nagao and colleagues also stated that the lunotriquetral ligament should be measured separately from the LTIO ligament.

Although Berger [17] did not find an attachment of the dorsal intercarpal ligament on the

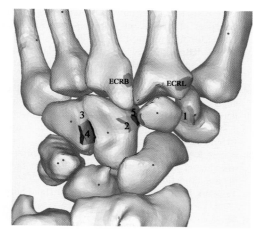

Fig. 11. A dorsal view of a 3-D model of a left wrist. The solid, colored areas show ligament attachment and the transparent colored areas show the paths of the ligaments. (*1*) Dorsal trapezium–trapezoid ligament. (*2*) Dorsal trapezoid–capitate ligament. (*3*) Dorsal capitate–hamate distal ligament. (*4*) Dorsal capitate–hamate proximal ligament. (*5*) Trapezoid–capitate interosseous ligament. ECRB, extensor carpi radialis brevis; ECRL, extensor carpi radialis longus.

lunate, Nagao and colleagues [3] found that the dorsal intercarpal ligament consistently attached to the lunate and that the dorsal intercarpal ligament had attachments dorsally on the triquetrum,

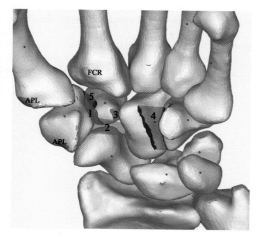

Fig. 12. A volarulnar view of a 3-D model of a left wrist. The solid, colored areas show ligament attachment and the transparent colored areas show the paths of the ligaments. (*1*) Volar trapezium–trapezoid ligament. (*2*) Volar trapezium–capitate ligament. (*3*) Volar trapezoid–capitate ligament. (*4*) Volar capitate–hamate ligament. (*5*) Trapezium–trapezoid interosseous ligament, APL, abductor pollicis longus; FCR, flexor carpi radialis.

lunate, proximal scaphoid, dorsal ridge at the waist of the scaphoid, and often on the trapezium [3]. Viegas and colleagues [25] previously described this anatomic variation of the dorsal intercarpal ligament. Based on this finding, Nagao and colleagues [3] suggested that the dorsal intercarpal ligament contributes to the stability of the entire proximal carpal row.

Summary

New and more detailed information on the skeletal morphology of the wrist and hand has been reported over the past 2 decades. This new information and better understanding of the ligament anatomy can help surgeons diagnose and treat the wrist, assess wrist images, and perform wrist arthroscopy. The recent work of Nagao and colleagues [3] and Nanno and colleagues [22,23] have shown the value of 3-D surface modeling in determining the specific locations and areas of ligament attachments of the distal radius, carpal, and metacarpal bones. Combining 3-D CT bone modeling with a 3-D depiction of the ligament attachments provides a better knowledge of the interrelation of the radiocarpal, carpal, and CMC ligaments and their attachments through visual illustration. These methods can also provide a better understanding of the pathomechanics in various wrist injuries, including injuries of the carpal ligaments. A more complete understanding of the anatomic location of the ligament attachments is important, particularly in their relation to the isometric points and kinematics of the carpal bones, the metacarpals, and ligament mechanics. This additional knowledge of the ligaments will help provide further understanding of wrist kinematics and, more precisely, the function of the individual ligaments and their roles in joint motion and stability and injuries.

Acknowledgments

The authors gratefully acknowledge the editorial assistance of Rebecca McGovney-Ingram during the preparation of this manuscript.

References

[1] Bettinger PC, Linscheid RL, Berger RA, et al. An anatomic study of the stabilizing ligaments of the trapezium and trapeziometacarpal joint. J Hand Surg [Am] 1999;24:786–98.

412

NANNO et al

[2] Nakamura K, Patterson RM, Viegas SF. The ligament and skeletal anatomy of the second through
fifth carpometacarpal joints and adjacent structures.
J Hand Surg [Am] 2001;26:1016–29.

[3] Nagao S, Patterson RM, Buford WL, et al. Three-
dimensional description of ligamentous attachments
around the lunate. J Hand Surg [Am] 2005;30:
685–92.

[4] Weitbrecht J. Syndesmology; or, a description of the
ligaments of the human body. Philadelphia: WB
Saunders; 1969 [Kaplan EB, Trans; original work
published 1742].

[5] Haines RW. The mechanism of rotation of the first
carpometacarpal joint. J Anat 1944;78:44–6.

[6] Napier JR. The form and function of the carpometacarpal joint of the thumb. J Anat 1955;89:
362–9.

[7] von Lanz T, Wachsmuth W. Praktische anatomie:
ein lehrund hilfsbuch der anatomischen grundlagen
ärztlichen Handelns. Berlin: Springer-Verlag; 1959.

[8] Kaplan EB, Riordan DC. The thumb. In:
Spinner M, editor. Kaplan's functional and surgical
anatomy of the hand. 3rd edition. Philadelphia: JB
Lippincott; 1984. p. 121–4.

[9] Pieron AP. The mechanism of the first carpometacarpal (CMC) joint. Acta Orthop Scand Suppl
1973;148:1–104.

[10] Pagalidis T, Kuczynski K, Lamb DW. Ligamentous
stability of the base of the thumb. Hand 1981;13:
29–35.

[11] Drewniany JJ, Palmer AK, Flatt AE. The scaphotrapezial ligament complex: an anatomic and biomechanical study. J Hand Surg [Am] 1985;10:492–8.

[12] Pellegrini VD. Osteoarthritis of the trapeziometacarpal joint: the pathophysiology of articular cartilage degeneration. I. Anatomy and pathology of
the aging joint. J Hand Surg [Am] 1991;16:967–74.

[13] Imaeda T, An K-N, Cooney WP III, et al. Anatomy
of trapeziometacarpal ligaments. J Hand Surg [Am]
1993;18:226–31.

[14] Harwin SF, Fox JM, Sedlin ED. Volar dislocation of
the bases of the second and third metacarpals.
J Bone Joint Surg [Am] 1975;57:849–51.

[15] Joseph RB, Linscheid RL, Dobyns JH, et al.
Chronic sprains of the carpometacarpal joints.
J Hand Surg [Am] 1981;6:172–80.

[16] Gurland M. Carpometacarpal joint injuries of the
fingers. Hand Clin 1992;8:733–44.

[17] Berger RA. The palmar radiocarpal ligaments:
a study of adult and fetal human wrist joints.
J Hand Surg [Am] 1990;15:847–54.

[18] Berger RA. The ligaments of the wrist: a current
overview of anatomy with considerations of their
potential functions. Hand Clin 1997;13:63–82.

[19] Taleisnik J. The ligaments of the wrist. J Hand Surg
[Am] 1976;1:110–8.

[20] Mayfield JK, Johnson RP, Kilcoyne RF. The ligaments of the wrist and their functional significance.
Anat Rec 1976;186:417–28.

[21] Viegas SF, Crossley M, Marzke M, et al. The fourth
carpometacarpal joint. J Hand Surg [Am] 1991;16:
525–33.

[22] Nanno M, Buford WL, Patterson RM, et al.
Three-dimensional analysis of ligamentous attachments of the carpometacarpal joints. The first carpometacarpal joint. Journal of Hand Surgery, in
press.

[23] Nanno M, Buford WL, Patterson RM, et al. Three-
dimensional analysis of ligamentous attachments of
the carpometacarpal joints. The second through
fifth carpometacarpal joints. Clinical Anatomy, in
press.

[24] Yoshida R, Shah MA, Patterson RM, et al. Anatomy and pathomechanics of ring and small finger
carpometacarpal joint injuries. J Hand Surg [Am]
2003;28:1035–43.

[25] Viegas SF, Yamaguchi S, Boyd NL, et al. The dorsal
ligaments of the wrist: anatomy, mechanical properties, and function. J Hand Surg [Am] 1999;24:
456–68.

ELSEVIER
SAUNDERS

Hand Clin 22 (2006) 413–420

HAND
CLINICS

Carpal Kinematics

Michael J. Gardner, MD[a], Joseph J. Crisco, PhD[b],
Scott W. Wolfe, MD[a],*

[a]Department of Orthopaedic Surgery, Hospital for Special Surgery, 535 East 70th Street, New York, NY 10021, USA
[b]Department of Orthopaedics, Brown Medical School/Rhode Island Hospital, Coro West, Suite 404,
1 Hoppin Street, Providence, RI 02903, USA

The motion of the eight carpal bones is extremely complex, and their accurate measurement has been hampered by their multiplanar rotations and translations, the irregularity of their shape, and the small magnitudes of movements. However, an accurate three-dimensional understanding of carpal motion is critical for academic and clinical purposes, and may play an important role in assessing surgical procedures or rehabilitation protocols.

Normal anatomic relationships and motion among the radius, scaphoid, and lunate are essential for normal wrist function [1]. Motion of the bones of the distal carpal row is initiated by the actions of the extrinsic wrist flexor and extensor tendons, and occurs at the midcarpal and radiocarpal articulations simultaneously. The proximal carpal row is an intercalated segment [2,3] whose direction of motion depends on the posture and movement of the distal carpal row, and whose stability and range depend on its ligamentous integrity and articular surface anatomy [4,5]. The scaphoid is the coordinating linkage between the proximal and distal carpal rows [6].

Kinematic analysis techniques

The study of carpal kinematics dates back to the late 19th century, soon after the discovery of x-rays, when Bryce [7] used plain radiographs to detail carpal motion in a cohort of normal subjects. Subsequent investigators have applied a multitude of techniques to study carpal motion, including anatomic dissections [8], cineradiography [9], stereoscopic radiography [10], and sonic digitization [11,12].

One proposed model for wrist function is the *column theory* of carpal motion [8]. Initially proposed by Navarro [13], the column theory organized the wrist into radial, central, and ulnar columns, based partially on phylogenetic data from birds and other species. Navarro surmised that, biomechanically, the capitolunate joint accommodated flexion–extension, the scaphoid stabilized the radial column, and the triquetriohamate joint allowed rotation. The three-column concept was redefined and popularized years later by Taleisnik [8].

Also around the turn of the 20th century, Etienne Destot led a surge of investigations using x-rays [14]. He encountered a sculptor with a fractured scaphoid, and this led to much research into carpal mechanics and mechanisms of carpal injuries [14]. He recognized the importance of the scapholunate ligament, and postulated that the bones of the wrist function as two independent rows [15]. Landsmeer [3] described the idea of the proximal row as an "intercalated segment," recognizing its balance between the fixed radius and the relatively rigid distal carpal row. This concept was further expanded to consider the two carpal rows as functionally distinct [12]. Whether the scaphoid is included as a member of the proximal row or is an independent link between the proximal and distal carpal rows is still debated [4,16].

Linscheid and colleagues [2] described another landmark concept of carpal kinematics, discussing posttraumatic collapse deformities relative to the

This article was funded in part by NIH AR44005.
* Corresponding author.
E-mail address: wolfes@hss.edu (S.W. Wolfe).

intercalated segment. The term *dorsal intercalated segment instability* (DISI) was coined to describe the typical dorsal lunate tilt posture associated with scapholunate pathology, whereas *volar intercalated segment instability* (VISI) identified the analogous condition related to lesions of the lunotriquetral joint [2].

Two decades later, Craigen and Stanley [17] used plain x-rays to study 52 wrists in vivo, and described two kinematic motion patterns of the scaphoid: one that moves predominantly in flexion–extension and one that moves principally in radioulnar deviation. Other authors have also noted this disparity [4,18], and one report correlated these different motion patterns with the degree of ligamentous laxity. The variability of carpal bone motion among subjects and the out-of-plane motions that occurred caused these and other authors to conclude that carpal kinematics was not uniform and, at least in the primary planes of wrist flexion–extension and radioulnar deviation, could not be inclusively described using either row or column theories.

Whether the inconsistencies among kinematic reports from different investigator teams were caused by true variability among subjects or by limitations in measurement techniques is of considerable debate. Using radiographs to describe the small multiplanar movements of the carpal bones has obvious limitations. Even with biplanar images, the complex morphology of the carpal bones makes quantifying their motion difficult, and specifically, rotation around the pronation–supination axis cannot be visualized. Recognition of the complex interdependent motion of the carpal bones in multiple planes spurred the development of three-dimensional analysis techniques.

In the past 25 years, many cadaveric models were developed using various techniques of carpal identification and tracking to measure three-dimensional motion [5,11,12,19–23]. Although much valuable information has been gained from these in vitro cadaveric kinematic studies, they have several inherent flaws. Most of these models use radio-opaque markers, rods, or other tracking devices, which inevitably interfere with the overlying soft tissues and extrinsic wrist ligaments and may alter the complex and sensitive normal kinematics. In addition, balanced muscle forces around the wrist have a significant impact on motion [21,24], and these are difficult to precisely simulate in cadaveric models.

Several authors used invasive marker systems in cadaveric in vitro studies to study pathologic states of the carpus [27–30]. Although these cadaver models allow specific and focal investigation of pathologies, their applicability to actual clinical conditions is also significantly limited because of the same restrictions. Sophisticated wrist simulator models were developed to study intact and simulated wrist injuries, and much information about the effect of ligament division and the impact of cyclic loading on carpal bone motion has been acquired using this technology [25]. True in vivo loads, however, cannot be properly ascertained for each condition, and therefore simulated forces in cadaveric studies are always approximations. Additionally, for unclear reasons, a hysteresis effect occurs in vivo, whereby dynamic carpal motion differs depending on the direction of motion [26]. An in vivo technique that would allow real-time visualization of carpal motion in intact and injured wrists would have several advantages, because actual muscle forces would be applied to move the wrist, and specific conditions and surgical treatments could be evaluated at serial time points in individual patients.

Delineation of detailed carpal kinematics with improved accuracy has paralleled technologic advances in imaging and computing. Recently, non-invasive markerless registration techniques using CT have been able to reproducibly register carpal bone position and accurately track carpal motion in three dimensions at different wrist positions [16,31–36]. The accuracy of one technique has been critically evaluated and found to be within 0.5° and 0.5 mm for the capitate and scaphoid motion, and 1.5° and 0.5 mm for the lunate [32].

One limitation of CT-based carpal kinematic registration is that it uses radiation, and therefore wrist motion must be imaged incrementally in quasi-static positions to limit radiation exposure, even when a low-dose scanning protocol is used [4,33,37]. To more closely approximate dynamic motion, a recent protocol used volume-based bone registration on MRI, thus eliminating radiation concerns and allowing smaller increments of motion to be studied [38]. This method combined surface and content image data to map and reconstruct the bones. Some authors believe that this technique may be less sensitive to segmentation errors than surface-based techniques [33], although other direct comparisons indicate that these two techniques have similar accuracy rates [32,38]. Despite the many studies that have attempted to explain carpal mechanics over the past hundred years, no unanimous theory or model fully explains wrist anatomy and function.

Anatomic motion planes

Most wrist kinematic studies have analyzed carpal bone behavior during wrist motion in the traditional anatomic planes: the sagittal plane (flexion-extension motion [FEM]) and the coronal plane (radioulnar deviation [RUD]). During wrist FEM, most studies have found that scaphoid motion occurs predominantly within the sagittal plane [11,21,22,25,26,39]. In FEM, the scaphoid and lunate follow the direction of wrist motion, but have less excursion because global wrist motion is composed of contributions from the distal and proximal rows [25]. In one study, scaphoid motion during wrist flexion equaled 73% of wrist motion and increased to 99% of wrist extension, whereas the lunate contributed only 46% of wrist flexion and 68% of wrist extension [16]. These findings indicate a significant amount of intercarpal motion between the scaphoid and lunate in normal wrist motion [16,21–23,39–41].

In the coronal plane of radial and ulnar wrist deviation, motion of the proximal carpal row has been more controversial [4,17,18]. One study reported that a subset of wrists showed scaphoid rotation primarily about the radioulnar deviation axis in the coronal plane [4]. However, our recent analysis using a highly accurate technique and a large number of subjects and wrist positions [32] concurred with previous studies [4,26,34] and found that scaphoid motion out of the FEM plane is minimal in all positions of wrist flexion, extension, and radial and ulnar deviation. Flexion and extension are associated with slight pronation and supination, respectively (average $1.9° \pm 2.8°$ arc), and slight scaphoid radial and ulnar deviation in wrist motion (average $1.7° \pm 3.1°$ arc) [39].

Qualitatively, lunate motion follows that of the scaphoid, and therefore moves almost entirely in the flexion–extension plane. In all positions of wrist motion, however, the magnitude of lunate motion is less than scaphoid motion [12,20,21, 38,39]. Using a three-dimensional volumetric MRI technique, Goto and colleagues [38] reported that the ratio of scaphoid motion to lunate motion in FEM was 1.43. These investigators found that the ratio of lunate motion to global wrist motion is constant, resulting in a linear relationship similar to the scaphoid. With full flexion of the wrist, 27% of the full flexion arc occurs between the scaphoid and lunate, which amounts to 16°. With full wrist extension, scapholunate motion similarly accounts for 27% of the extension arc,

and quantitatively 19° of motion occurs at the scapholunate joint [16].

The recent development of precise in vivo analysis techniques has also allowed investigators to identify and quantify small translational moments of the carpus. The scaphoid translates in the range of 2 to 4 mm, and occurs almost completely in the radial direction. The lunate also translates radially, but less so than the scaphoid [39]. The coupled extension and radial translation of the scaphoid and lunate is consistent with the original "screw-home" theory as a component of normal carpal motion [42].

In contrast to the proximal carpal row, the distal carpal bones have a more constant relationship with each other. The capitate is anatomically situated such that it has been considered the keystone of the wrist [11,22], although some investigators have disagreed about capitate motion and the center of rotation of the wrist. Savelberg and colleagues [43] reported that the wrist pivoted around a single transverse axis centered in the proximal pole of the capitate, implying that the wrist functions as a single joint. Using high-speed video acquisition and CT reconstructions, Patterson and colleagues [40] concluded that the wrist may not flex and extend around a single axis of rotation.

Using an in vivo, three-dimensional, CT-based method, Neu and colleagues [44] recently showed that with wrist flexion, the capitate undergoes minor degrees of complex multiplanar motion, including flexion, pronation, ulnar deviation, and slight ulnar translation. With wrist extension, the capitate moves in opposite directions, except that it also undergoes ulnar deviation with extension. With radial deviation, the main motion of the capitate is in extension, whereas with wrist ulnar deviation, the main plane of capitate motion is ulnar deviation (Fig. 1). The center of rotation of the capitate is not constant throughout the range of motion, and depends particularly on the degree of flexion and ulnar deviation. The axes of capitate rotation shift depending on position and do not intersect at a single point, indicating that the wrist does not act as a universal pivot joint and instead moves through multiple and complex mechanisms. However, the capitate rotation axes shift only by approximately 4 mm, so a single pivot point of the capitate is a reasonable assumption for studies that consider global wrist motion on a larger scale. Finally, the capitate and the third metacarpal are essentially rigid and move as a single unit throughout the entire wrist motion range

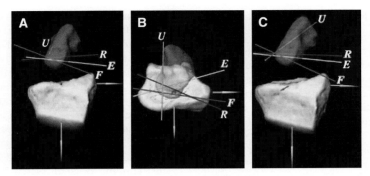

Fig. 1. Typical capitate motion axes in flexion (F), extension (E), ulnar deviation (U), and radial deviation (R) are shown in a coronal (A), proximal (B), and oblique (C) view. The motion axes do not intersect at a single point in the proximal capitate, showing that the wrist does not move about a single point like a universal joint and that different carpal mechanisms exist through which wrist flexion, extension, radial deviation, and ulnar deviation occur. (*From* Neu CP, Crisco JJ, Wolfe SW. In vivo kinematic behavior of the radio-capitate joint during wrist flexion-extension and radio-ulnar deviation. J Biomech 2001;34:1429–38; with permission.)

[23,39,40,44]. This constant relationship allows radiocapitate motion to be used as an indicator of global wrist motion, and simplifies visualization of carpal kinematics by equating hand posture in space with the position of the capitate, relative to a fixed radial coordinate system [16].

Historic models of scaphotrapezio–trapezoid (STT) joint motion show that negligible motion occurs between the trapezium and trapezoid, and that this rigid complex articulates with the scaphoid along a single path from radial-extension to flexion-ulnar deviation through the interfacet ridge [45,46]. However, these conclusions were based on data from a cadaver model, which may not have been sensitive enough to detect small amounts of motion. An in vivo analysis has more recently shown that although less movement occurs between the trapezium and trapezoid than between other carpal articulations, they do not move strictly as a single unit (Fig. 2) [35]. Although the trapezium and trapezoid generally both move as a unit relative to the scaphoid, this movement depends on the direction of motion, and they do not move only along a single path for all ranges of motion. During wrist flexion, the trapezoid travels with the capitate, whereas the trapezium flexes to a lesser degree and may be tethered by the lagging scaphoid flexion.

The dart thrower's motion

Considerable controversy remains and conflicting reports exist regarding carpal bone motion in the traditional planes of FEM and RUD. Although some of the discrepancy may be related to variations in measurement techniques and anatomic variability among human subjects, no clear unifying theory has explained carpal kinematics in the planes of flexion–extension and radioulnar deviation. The vision of carpal kinematics may be obscured by the constraint of carpal motion into arbitrary and orthogonal planes of motion. In fact, most functional activities involve combined motions of flexion–ulnar deviation and extension–radial deviation: the so-called "dart-thrower's plane" of motion [20,25,38,39,47]. Dart thrower's motion (DTM) involves an obliquely oriented plane of wrist motion that ranges from positions of combined radial deviation and extension to positions of combined ulnar deviation and flexion. This motion is used in many daily and recreational activities, including combing the hair, wringing a washcloth, tying a shoelace, pouring from a pitcher, hammering nails, throwing objects, and swinging a bat or golf club, and others that require a combination of strength and fine motor control [47]. This motion path is believed to not only provide more agility and mobility [48,49] but also confer a degree of inherent stability that allows for a sustained power grip during motion.

Despite the perceived relative importance of this wrist motion, its kinematic nuances have only rarely been reported. Saffar and Seemaan [49] noted that during wrist motion in this plane, most carpal motion occurs at the midcarpal joint in an oblique plane with no rotational shift of the proximal carpal row. Using a cadaveric model and a magnetic tracking device coupled with wrist distraction to evaluate DTM, Ishikawa and

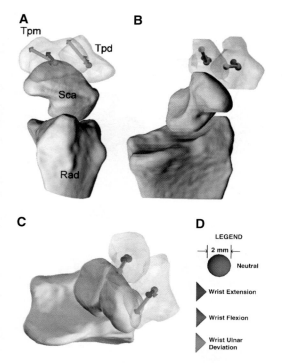

A
Tpm
B
Tpd
Sca
Rad

C
D
LEGEND
2 mm
Neutral
Wrist Extension
Wrist Flexion
Wrist Ulnar Deviation

Fig. 2. Average centroid displacements show that the trapezoid and trapezium follow similar ulnar–flexion paths with respect to the scaphoid. The average displacements (*solid arrows*) of trapezoid and trapezium centroids from neutral (*purple sphere*) to wrist motions of $40° \pm 10°$ were significantly greater in wrist ulnar deviation (*green*) than in wrist extension (*blue*) or flexion (*red*). The radius (Rad), scaphoid (Sca), trapezoid (Tpd), and trapezium (Tpm) of a right wrist in a typical neutral position in a radial (*A*), palmar (*B*), and proximal (*C*) view. Although the scale varies throughout this figure, the diameter of the neutral centroid always represents 2 mm (*D*). (*From* Sonenblum SE, Crisco JJ, Kang L, et al. In vivo motion of the scaphotrapezio-trapezoidal (STT) joint. J Biomech 2004;37:645–52; with permission.)

colleagues [20] reported that relative scapholunate motion was more unified and generally decreased in this plane, and that the dart thrower's plane probably represents a more physiologic motion path.

The scaphoid extends with wrist extension and flexes with radial deviation. Therefore, at some intermediate angle between full extension and radial deviation, the scaphoid position is neutral and remains so as the wrist returns to neutral. One cadaver study tracked scaphoid and lunate motion with seven intermediate motion paths between pure FEM and RUD, finding that the

transition between scaphoid flexion and extension occurs between 10° and 15° off of the sagittal plane along the dart thrower's path. The transition point for the lunate occurs between 10° and 20° [25]. Moreover, during wrist motion along this path of radial extension to ulnar flexion, the scaphoid and the lunate contribute as little as 22% to 26% of total wrist motion [25]. However, these studies evaluated carpal kinematics along predetermined motion paths that were difficult to quantify.

A recent in vivo study from our institutions specifically analyzed carpal motion during DTM [39]. This analysis involved creating a large database of CT images of multiple wrist positions and deriving the carpal positions post hoc, which allowed for more accurate interpolation compared with analysis at predetermined wrist positions. The best-fit plane that fit neutral scaphoid rotation was oriented obliquely, thus the intersection with zero scaphoid flexion–extension rotation resulted in an oblique line that fell along the dart thrower's path. This path passes approximately through neutral wrist position. The motion path that corresponds to zero lunate rotation also lies obliquely from radial extension to ulnar flexion but, interestingly, is not exactly coincident with that of the scaphoid, and differs by approximately 10° (Fig. 3).

Clinical implications

The clear and comprehensive derivation of normal carpal kinematics has potentially significant implications in pathologic and postsurgical states. For example, to evaluate the effects of external fixation and traction on carpal kinematics, Ishikawa and colleagues [20] applied a cadaver model that was used previously to study normal wrist kinematics. They found that wrist extension under traction had a greater effect on the proximal radiocarpal ligaments, which limited scaphoid and overall wrist extension relative to the midcarpal joint. This effect was opposite in flexion, during which radiocarpal motion increased and midcarpal motion decreased with traction. Therefore, distraction, which is often a necessary component of closed reduction and external fixation of distal radius fractures, tightens the carpal ligaments differentially and leads to abnormal carpal kinematics [20]. Patterson and colleagues [50] applied three different dynamic external fixators across the wrist joint that were designed to allow wrist motion around an axis through the capitate.

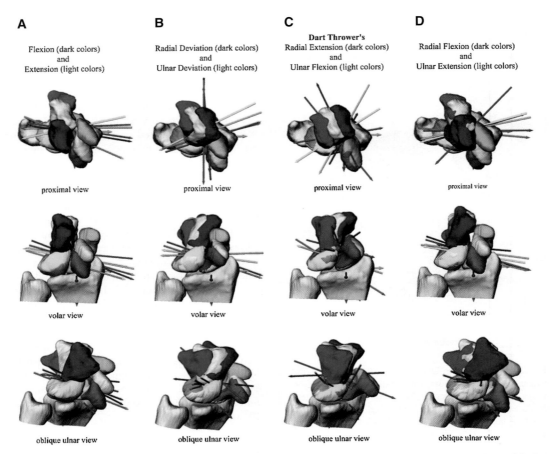

A

Flexion (dark colors)
and
Extension (light colors)

proximal view

volar view

oblique ulnar view

B

Radial Deviation (dark colors)
and
Ulnar Deviation (light colors)

proximal view

volar view

oblique ulnar view

C

Dart Thrower's
Radial Extension (dark colors)
and
Ulnar Flexion (light colors)

proximal view

volar view

oblique ulnar view

D

Radial Flexion (dark colors)
and
Ulnar Extension (light colors)

proximal view

volar view

oblique ulnar view

Fig. 3. Three views of the scaphoid, lunate, capitate, and distal parts of the radius and ulna in wrist positions of flexion and extension (*A*), radial and ulnar deviation (*B*), dart thrower's radial extension and ulnar flexion (*C*), and radial flexion and ulnar extension (*D*). The bones in their neutral position are colored gray. The rotation axes for the motion of the scaphoid, lunate, and capitate from neutral to each respective position are colored similar to the corresponding carpal bone. The minimal rotation of the scaphoid and lunate in the dart thrower's positions (*C*) can be seen best in the volar and oblique views. (*From* Crisco JJ, Coburn JC, Moore DC, et al. In vivo radiocarpal kinematics and the dart thrower's motion. J Bone Joint Surg Am 2005;87:2729–40; with permission.)

They confirmed that the axis of normal wrist motion is not static or centered in the capitate, and that the dynamic external fixators tested did not permit normal carpal motion.

Further refinement of the DTM path and its effect on carpal kinematics will likely significantly impact pathologic disorders and rehabilitation protocols. A distinct motion path exists from radial deviation/extension to ulnar deviation/flexion, which is the transition point between scaphoid and lunate flexion and extension [39]. Limiting wrist motion to this path would minimize motion of the scaphoid and lunate and their articulations, allowing early mobilization and prevention of

stiffness while protecting arthrodeses, ligament repairs, and fracture stabilization [25].

Summary

Understanding of the complex intercarpal motion that occurs with wrist motion has greatly advanced over the past century, largely because of the multitude of in vitro studies that laid the groundwork for carpal kinematics and the more recent development of noninvasive, markerless in vivo CT and MRI techniques for precisely measuring carpal mechanics. Because these newer techniques are still in their infancy, they have not yielded a unified theory on wrist motion. As collaborative research continues, important information on carpal motion in normal and pathologic states will inevitably be obtained, potentially leading to improved evaluations for lesions of the wrist and better outcomes instruments for surgical procedures.

References

[1] Garcia-Elias M, Cooney WP, An KN, et al. Wrist kinematics after limited intercarpal arthrodesis. J Hand Surg [Am] 1989;14:791–9.

[2] Linscheid RL, Dobyns JH, Beabout JW, et al. Traumatic instability of the wrist. Diagnosis, classification, and pathomechanics. J Bone Joint Surg Am 1972;54:1612–32.

[3] Landsmeer JM. Studies in the anatomy of articulation. I. The equilibrium of the "intercalated" bone. Acta Morphol Neerl Scand 1961;3:287–303.

[4] Moojen TM, Snel JG, Ritt MJ, et al. Scaphoid kinematics in vivo. J Hand Surg [Am] 2002;27:1003–10.

[5] Horii E, An KN, Linscheid RL. Excursion of prime wrist tendons. J Hand Surg [Am] 1993;18:83–90.

[6] Linscheid RL. Kinematic considerations of the wrist. Clin Orthop Relat Res 1986;(202):27–39.

[7] Bryce TH. On certain points in the anatomy and mechanism of the wrist-joint reviewed in light of a series of Roentgen ray photographs of the living hand. J Anat Physiol 1896;31:59.

[8] Taleisnik J. The ligaments of the wrist. J Hand Surg [Am] 1976;1:110–8.

[9] Arkless R. Cineradiography in normal and abnormal wrists. Am J Roentgenol Radium Ther Nucl Med 1966;96:837.

[10] Wright RD. A detailed study of movement of the wrist joint. J Anat 1970;70:137.

[11] Ruby LK, Cooney WP III, An KN, et al. Relative motion of selected carpal bones: a kinematic analysis of the normal wrist. J Hand Surg [Am] 1988;13:1–10.

[12] Berger RA, Crowninshield RD, Flatt AE. The three-dimensional rotational behaviors of the carpal bones. Clin Orthop Relat Res 1982;(167):303–10.

[13] Navarro A. Luxaciones del carpo. An Fac Med (Lima) 1921;6:113–41.

[14] Dobyns JH, Linscheid RL. A short history of the wrist joint. Hand Clin 1997;13:1–12.

[15] Destot E. Injuries of the wrist: a radiological study. New York: Paul B. Hoeber; 1926 [Atkinson FRB, Trans.]

[16] Wolfe SW, Neu C, Crisco JJ. In vivo scaphoid, lunate, and capitate kinematics in flexion and in extension. J Hand Surg [Am] 2000;25:860–9.

[17] Craigen MA, Stanley JK. Wrist kinematics. Row, column or both? J Hand Surg [Br] 1995;20:165–70.

[18] Garcia-Elias M, Ribe M, Rodriguez J, et al. Influence of joint laxity on scaphoid kinematics. J Hand Surg [Br] 1995;20:379–82.

[19] Gellman H, Kauffman D, Lenihan M, et al. An in vitro analysis of wrist motion: the effect of limited intercarpal arthrodesis and the contributions of the radiocarpal and midcarpal joints. J Hand Surg [Am] 1988;13:378–83.

[20] Ishikawa J, Cooney WP III, Niebur G, et al. The effects of wrist distraction on carpal kinematics. J Hand Surg [Am] 1999;24:113–20.

[21] Kobayashi M, Berger RA, Nagy L, et al. Normal kinematics of carpal bones: a three-dimensional analysis of carpal bone motion relative to the radius. J Biomech 1997;30:787–93.

[22] Savelberg HH, Kooloos JG, De Lange A, et al. Human carpal ligament recruitment and three-dimensional carpal motion. J Orthop Res 1991;9:693–704.

[23] Werner FW, Short WH, Fortino MD, et al. The relative contribution of selected carpal bones to global wrist motion during simulated planar and out-of-plane wrist motion. J Hand Surg [Am] 1997;22:708–13.

[24] Valero-Cuevas FJ, Small CF. Load dependence in carpal kinematics during wrist flexion in vivo. Clin Biomech (Bristol, Avon) 1997;12:154–9.

[25] Werner FW, Green JK, Short WH, et al. Scaphoid and lunate motion during a wrist dart throw motion. J Hand Surg [Am] 2004;29:418–22.

[26] Short WH, Werner FW, Fortino MD, et al. Analysis of the kinematics of the scaphoid and lunate in the intact wrist joint. Hand Clin 1997;13:93–108.

[27] Smith DK, An KN, Cooney WP III, et al. Effects of a scaphoid waist osteotomy on carpal kinematics. J Orthop Res 1989;7:590–8.

[28] Short WH, Werner FW, Fortino MD, et al. A dynamic biomechanical study of scapholunate ligament sectioning. J Hand Surg [Am] 1995;20:986–99.

[29] Ruby LK, An KN, Linscheid RL, et al. The effect of scapholunate ligament section on scapholunate motion. J Hand Surg [Am] 1987;12:767–71.

[30] Dagum AB, Hurst LC, Finzel KC. Scapholunate dissociation: an experimental kinematic study of two types of indirect soft tissue repairs. J Hand Surg [Am] 1997;22:714–9.

[31] Feipel V, Rooze M. Three-dimensional motion patterns of the carpal bones: an in vivo study using three-dimensional computed tomography and clinical applications. Surg Radiol Anat 1999;21:125–31.

[32] Neu CP, McGovern RD, Crisco JJ. Kinematic accuracy of three surface registration methods in a three-dimensional wrist bone study. J Biomech Eng 2000;122:528–33.

[33] Moojen TM, Snel JG, Ritt MJ, et al. In vivo analysis of carpal kinematics and comparative review of the literature. J Hand Surg [Am] 2003;28:81–7.

[34] Moojen TM, Snel JG, Ritt MJ, et al. Three-dimensional carpal kinematics in vivo. Clin Biomech (Bristol, Avon) 2002;17:506–14.

[35] Sonenblum SE, Crisco JJ, Kang L, et al. In vivo motion of the scaphotrapezio-trapezoidal (STT) joint. J Biomech 2004;37:645–52.

[36] Crisco JJ, McGovern RD, Wolfe SW. Noninvasive technique for measuring in vivo three-dimensional carpal bone kinematics. J Orthop Res 1999;17: 96–100.

[37] Snel JG, Venema HW, Moojen TM, et al. Quantitative in vivo analysis of the kinematics of carpal bones from three-dimensional CT images using a deformable surface model and a three-dimensional matching technique. Med Phys 2000;27:2037–47.

[38] Goto A, Moritomo H, Murase T, et al. In vivo three-dimensional wrist motion analysis using magnetic resonance imaging and volume-based registration. J Orthop Res 2005;23:750–6.

[39] Crisco JJ, Coburn JC, Moore DC, et al. In vivo radiocarpal kinematics and the dart thrower's motion. J Bone Joint Surg Am 2005;87:2729–40.

[40] Patterson RM, Nicodemus CL, Viegas SF, et al. High-speed, three-dimensional kinematic analysis of the normal wrist. J Hand Surg [Am] 1998;23: 446–53.

[41] Short WH, Werner FW, Green JK, et al. Biomechanical evaluation of ligamentous stabilizers of the scaphoid and lunate. J Hand Surg [Am] 2002; 27:991–1002.

[42] McConaill MA. The mechanical anatomy of the carpus and its bearing on some surgical problems. J Anat 1941;75:166–75.

[43] Savelberg HH, Otten JD, Kooloos JG, et al. Carpal bone kinematics and ligament lengthening studied for the full range of joint movement. J Biomech 1993;26:1389–402.

[44] Neu CP, Crisco JJ, Wolfe SW. In vivo kinematic behavior of the radio-capitate joint during wrist flexion-extension and radio-ulnar deviation. J Biomech 2001;34:1429–38.

[45] Moritomo H, Viegas SF, Elder K, et al. The scapho-trapezio-trapezoidal joint. Part 2: a kinematic study. J Hand Surg [Am] 2000;25:911–20.

[46] Kauer JM. The mechanism of the carpal joint. Clin Orthop Relat Res 1986;(202):16–26.

[47] Palmer AK, Werner FW, Murphy D, et al. Functional wrist motion: a biomechanical study. J Hand Surg [Am] 1985;10:39–46.

[48] Li ZM, Kuxhaus L, Fisk JA, et al. Coupling between wrist flexion-extension and radial-ulnar deviation. Clin Biomech (Bristol, Avon) 2005;20:177–83.

[49] Saffar P, Seemaan I. The study of biomechanics of wrist movements in an oblique plane. A preliminary report. In: Schiund F, An KN, Cooney WP III, et al, editors. Advances in the biomechanics of the hand and wrist. New York: Plenum Press; 1994. p. 305–11.

[50] Patterson RM, Nicodemus CL, Viegas SF, et al. Normal wrist kinematics and the analysis of the effect of various dynamic external fixators for treatment of distal radius fractures. Hand Clin 1997;13: 129–41.

ELSEVIER
SAUNDERS

Hand Clin 22 (2006) 421–434

Surgical Approaches to the Carpus

Shian Chao Tay, MD[a,b], Alexander Y. Shin, MD[a]

[a]*Department of Orthopaedic Surgery, Division of Hand Surgery, Mayo Clinic College of Medicine,*
200 First Street SW, Rochester, MN 55905, USA
[b]*Department of Hand Surgery, Singapore General Hospital, Outram Road, Singapore 169608*

Nowhere else in the body are the general principles of surgical exposures—which include adequate access, extensibility, preservation of vital structures, minimizing collateral tissue trauma (to reduce the healing load), maximizing primary wound healing, and cosmesis—more applicable than in the hand and wrist. Because the relation of deeper structures is very intimate in the hand, protection and prevention of injury to vital structures, such as important ligaments, tendons, nerves and vessels, is very important. The sensory function of the hand represents one of the largest portions of the sensory homunculus [1]. As such, preservation of sensory nerves is paramount to prevent creation of painful neuromas that may result in a painful wound, which may be so severe as to cause the patient to alienate his hand [2,3], sabotaging the purpose of the surgical procedure. The design of the skin incision must take into account the relation of deeper structures, the sensory distribution of the area being exposed (to avoid damage to the sensory nerves and its branches), the presence of flexion creases (to avoid skin and joint contractures), the vascular supply to the skin or skin flaps, the presence of previous wounds, and finally, cosmesis. A keen knowledge of anatomy is paramount in understanding and applying the surgical approaches for the wrist.

Carpal exposures can be divided into general exposures and specific exposures. General exposures provide wide exposure to large areas of the wrist, including the radiocarpal joint, midcarpal joint, and intercarpal joints, and allow for access to pathology that may involving multiple joints or multiple carpal bones.

Specific approaches give access to a single bone or joint for management of a discrete condition, and usually have only one purpose. As a result,

they provide limited exposure and may not be easily extensible. They should be reserved for situations where the diagnosis is clear and the management is precise.

Dorsal carpal exposure: general

The dorsal carpal exposure is one of the most important general approaches to the carpus, because it gives the surgeon more options and substantially more exposure than the palmar approaches. This is because of the relative paucity of extrinsic ligaments on the dorsum of the carpus compared with the volar carpus. There are essentially two dorsal ligaments that are intimate with the dorsal capsule: the dorsal radiocarpal (radiotriquetral) ligament, and the dorsal intercarpal (scaphotriquetral) ligament (Fig. 1) [4–6]. Previous descriptions of capsular incisions included a longitudinal incision that divided the dorsal radiocarpal and intercarpal ligaments; however, a dorsal capsulotomy that exploits the dorsal ligaments was described by Berger and colleagues [6,7]. In their ligament-sparing capsulotomy, the dorsal intercarpal and radiocarpal ligaments were divided in line with the fibers, and a radial-based flap of capsule was created, providing excellent exposure to the entire carpus (Fig. 2). Variations of this approach will allow the surgeon access to the radiocarpal joint, midcarpal joint, ulnocarpal joint, or all of the above.

Skin and subcutaneous tissue

The wrist and forearm are placed into a neutral rotation position, and a line is drawn centered about the third metacarpal, extending proximally (Fig. 3). The length of the incision is dependant on

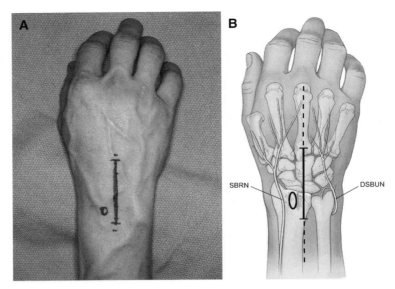

Fig. 1. (*A*) Dorsal exposure of the carpus can be accomplished through either transverse or longitudinal. The extensile nature of the longitudinal incision is favored over the transverse incision. The longitudinal incision (*solid line*) is centered about the third metacarpal and is ulnar to Lister's tubercle (*oval*). A 3–6 cm incision is used to expose the carpus and can be extended as needed (*dotted line*). (*B*) Diagrammatic representation of the skin incision, showing its relations to the third metacarpal, Lister's tubercle, and the dorsal cutaneous branches of the radial and ulnar nerve. DSBUN, dorsal sensory branch of the ulnar nerve; SBRN, superficial branch of the radial nerve. (*A* and *B* copyright 2006 Mayo Clinics, reproduced with permission of the Mayo Foundation.)

the surgery performed. The authors do not particularly recommend curvilinear or zigzag incisions, because they do not appreciably improve either the exposure or the cosmesis of the wound scar.

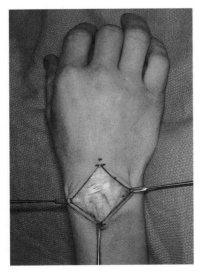

Fig. 2. Under brachial tourniquet control, full-thickness skin flaps are elevated and the transverse fibers of the extensor retinaculum are exposed.

Furthermore, there is a risk of flap ischemia or necrosis with curvilinear or zigzag incisions, particularly in patients who have poor skin vascularity [8,9]. The other important consideration of this incision is that it will most likely avoid the branches of the superficial radial nerve and the dorsal cutaneous branch of the ulnar nerve [10–14]. If distal extension of the incision is required beyond the base of the third metacarpal, one should be wary of the more ulnar branches of the superficial radial nerve [14].

Full-thickness flaps containing the skin, subcutaneous tissues, and superficial fascia should be raised together to expose the extensor retinaculum (see Fig. 2). Large longitudinal veins should be preserved, but crossing branches can be divided. The dorsal sensory branches of the radial and ulnar nerve should remain in the flaps and be preserved and protected (Fig. 4). It is often the authors' practice to identify the sensory nerves, and if necessary, place vessel loops around them to protect them.

Retinaculum

Starting just ulnar to Lister's tubercle, the course of the extensor pollicis longus is identified and the third dorsal compartment opened (Fig. 5).

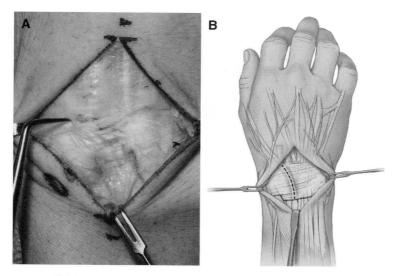

Fig. 3. (*A*) The extensor pollicis longus tendon at the distal margin of the extensor retinaculum is identified (*probe*) and the course of the extensor pollicis longus is determined. (*B*) The incision on the extensor retinaculum (*dashed line*) is designed over the extensor pollicis longus tendon. (Copyright 2006 Mayo Clinics, reproduced with permission of the Mayo Foundation.)

The proximal and distal extent of the extensor retinaculum [15] should then be identified (Fig. 6) and the retinaculum elevated ulnarly by dividing the septum between the third and fourth, and fourth and fifth extensor compartments (Fig. 7). The authors have found that preserving the integrity of the fourth dorsal compartment is not critical, and thus we do not perform subperiosteal dissection of that compartment any more. To gain full exposure of the dorsal carpus, the retinacular flap should be carried ulnarward to the fifth extensor compartment. It is imperative that in performing this, the extensor retinaculum not be detached inadvertently. It is easiest to identify

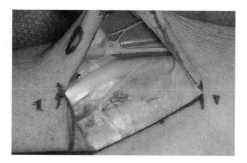

Fig. 4. Preservation of the branches of the superficial branch of the radial nerve are important. They are located radial to the extensor pollicus longus tendon, and often have branches that can course over it.

the extensor digiti minimi proximally, which will facilitate division of the fifth compartment from the radial side. The extensor pollicis longus tendon should be retracted radially with the extensor carpi radialis tendons, and the extensor digitorum communis, extensor indicis proprius, and extensor digiti minimi tendons should be retracted ulnarly. Once this is done, the floors of the third, fourth, and fifth compartments are exposed, exposing the dorsal wrist capsule and its ligaments (Fig. 8). At the radial margin of the fourth compartment lies the posterior interosseous nerve. It is routinely resected for pain relief as part of this exposure [16,17].

Capsule

The ligament-sparing approach uses a capsulotomy that splits the fibers of the dorsal radiocarpal and dorsal intercarpal ligaments. The required landmarks are the dorsal radiocarpal ligament, dorsal intercarpal ligament, dorsal tubercle of the triquetrum (where the dorsal intercarpal ligament and dorsal radiocarpal ligament attach), and the scaphoid. The width of the dorsal radiocarpal ligament is estimated, and it is bisected sharply through a fiber-splitting division down the middle of the ligament from the radius to the triquetrum. Care it taken not to injure the underlying structures (cartilage or ligaments). The radial start point is roughly halfway between Lister's tubercle and the

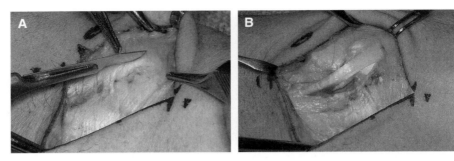

Fig. 5. (*A*) The third extensor compartment is opened, and (*B*) the extensor pollicis longus tendon is exposed (*distal is the right side of the photograph*).

sigmoid notch. In a similar fashion, beginning at the dorsal tubercle of the triquetrum, the dorsal intercarpal ligament is sharply bisected until its attachment to the scaphoid is reached. The midpoint of the attachment of the dorsal intercarpal ligament is approximately at the junction between the distal scaphoid and the trapezoid. Care should be taken here not to disrupt the dorsal vascular supply of the scaphoid. The capsulotomy is then elevated from the triquetrum and advanced radially and proximally until the dorsal rim of the radius is reached. The capsulotomy is completed by radial extension along the dorsal rim of the distal radius, leaving a rim of tissue for subsequent repair (Fig. 9). Care should be taken during the elevation of this

capsular flap not to injure the scapholunate ligament and the lunotriquetral ligaments, which are intimately related to the capsular flap as it is being raised [4,5,15,18]. When approaching these structures, the scalpel blade has to be angled sufficiently to skive over the dorsal surfaces of the respective intercarpal joints and the dorsal surfaces of the proximal carpal bones to release capsule, and not the interosseous ligaments.

Exposure

This capsulotomy will allow exposure of the radiocarpal joint, proximal scaphoid, lunate, and

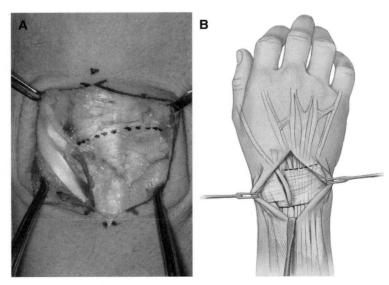

Fig. 6. (*A*) The proximal and the distal extentd of the extensor retinaculum are identified and carefully incised as shown (*dashed line*). Care must be taken to not inadvertently injure the extensor tendons beneath the retinaculum. The ulnarmost aspect of the transverse incision of the retinaculum is carried to the fifth extensor compartment. (*B*) A diagrammatic representation of the distal retinacular incision (*dashed line*). (Copyright 2006 Mayo Clinics, reproduced with permission of the Mayo Foundation.)

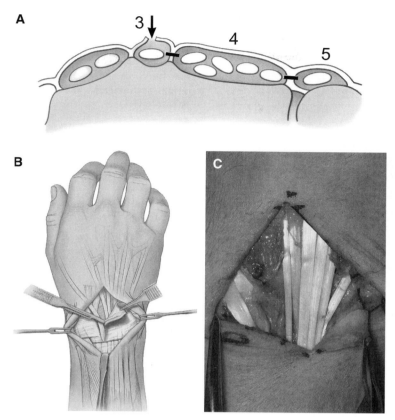

Fig. 7. (*A*) Elevation of the retinacular flap is performed by dividing the septum between the third and fourth, and fourth and fifth extensor compartments (*dashes*) after exposing the 3rd compartment (*arrow*). This drawing shows a cross-sectional view through the extensor retinaculum. It is not necessary to perform a subperiosteal dissection, only to divide the septation between the third and fourth, and fourth and fifth compartments. (*B*) The extensor retinaculum is elevated in a radial-to-ulnar direction after making the proximal and distal retinacular incisions. Care must be taken not to injure the extensor tendons. (*C*) On completion of the retinacular flap, the tendons of the third, fourth and fifth extensor compartments are exposed and an ulnar based retinacular flap is created. (*A* and *B* copyright 2006 Mayo Clinics, reproduced with permission of the Mayo Foundation.)

parts of the capitate, hamate, and triquetrum. (Fig. 10).

Modifications

Further radial extension can be achieved by elevating the extensor retinaculum off Lister's tubercle, as a radial retinacular flap exposing the second extensor compartment. Osteotomy of Lister's tubercle is no longer routinely performed. This effectively releases the second compartment tendons, allowing greater radial retraction of the extensor carpi radialis brevis and longus for the dorsal capsulotomy to be extended more radially.

If exposure of the ulnocarpal joint is required instead of the radiocarpal joint, a capsulotomy

with a proximally based capsular flap should be used instead (Fig. 11A) [6]. The landmarks for this capsular flap are the dorsal tubercle of the triquetrum, the dorsal radioulnar ligament, and the dorsal radiocarpal ligament. The width of the dorsal radiocarpal ligament is estimated, and it is bisected roughly from a point midway between Lister's tubercle and the sigmoid notch, to the dorsal tubercle of the triquetrum, in a fiber-splitting fashion. Immediately deep to the sixth dorsal compartment, the capsulotomy is advanced proximally in longitudinal fashion until the dorsal radioulnar ligament is reached. This marks the proximal extent of the capsulotomy. The triangular fibrocartilage complex, proximal surfaces of

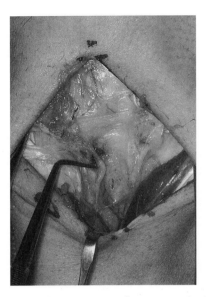

Fig. 8. With the extensor tendons appropriately re-tracted, the dorsal wrist capsule and ligaments are ex-posed. The posterior interosseous nerve is typically found lying on the floor of the radial side of the fourth extensor compartment. It runs distally and innervates the dorsal wrist capsule. It is typically divided and a seg-ment discarded.

the lunate and triquetrum, and the lunotriquetral ligament will be visible (Fig. 11B).

If exposure of the midcarpal joint is required, a distally based capsulotomy can be performed [6]. The landmarks for this include the triquetrum, the scaphoid, and the dorsal intercarpal ligament. Again, the width of the dorsal intercarpal liga-ment is estimated, and it is bisected sharply down its middle in a fiber-splitting fashion from the triquetrum to the scaphoid. The flap is then elevated from the triquetrum and reflected dis-tally, leaving the capsular attachments to scaph-oid intact. The midcarpal joint will be exposed with the distal articular surfaces of the scaphoid, lunate, and triquetrum, and the proximal surfaces of the trapezium, trapezoid, capitate, and hamate.

Rarely, the entire carpus might need to be exposed. A dorsal pan-carpal capsulotomy can be performed in a manner to maximally maintain ligamentous integrity. The proximal edge of the dorsal radiocarpal ligament and the distal edge of the dorsal intercarpal ligament are identified (usually at the level of the carpometacarpal joint), and an incision along these borders is made. A small osteotome is then used to elevate the dorsal

cortex of the triquetrum, leaving the common attachments of the dorsal radiocarpal ligament and the dorsal intercarpal ligament intact. This bone-ligament-capsular flap is then reflected radi-ally until the scaphoid is reached. The radial origin of the dorsal radiocarpal ligament can be separated, but a small rim of tissue should be left on the radius to allow subsequent repair. This capsulotomy will allow complete exposure of the radiocarpal joint, the ulnocarpal joint, and the midcarpal joint.

Closure

The radially based dorsal capsular flap is replaced, and the dorsal radiocarpal and dorsal intercarpal ligaments are reapposed using absorb-able sutures (Fig. 12). If a proximally based ulnar flap was created for ulnocarpal exposure, closure is easily done by repair of the flap to the dorsal radiocarpal ligament. The distally based midcar-pal capsulotomy can also be similarly repaired to the dorsal intercarpal ligament with sutures.

If a pan-carpal capsulotomy is performed, a stout repair of the radial origin of the dorsal radiocarpal ligament needs to be done to the rim of tissue or via intraosseous suture anchors. The dorsal triquetral cortex is secured by a standard small cortical screw, thereby anchoring the ulnar attachments of the dorsal radiocarpal and dorsal intercarpal ligaments.

Following capsular repair, the extensor ten-dons except the extensor pollicis longus are replaced in their original positions, and the radial and ulnar retinacular flaps are repaired directly to each other using interrupted absorbable sutures. The extensor pollicis longus is routinely dorsally transposed.

Volar carpal exposure: carpal tunnel approach

There are essentially two types of volar carpal exposures, one that divides the transverse carpal ligament and one that uses a modified Henry approach. The volar carpal exposure is most commonly used to reduce difficult carpal disloca-tions (perilunar) and for repair or reconstruction of the palmar wrist capsule and the palmar carpal ligaments. Volar approaches are also useful for reduction and fixation of palmar fragments of difficult distal radius fractures. The volar ap-proach is often used in combination with a dorsal approach in the management of the Mayfield type of carpal injuries [19–21].

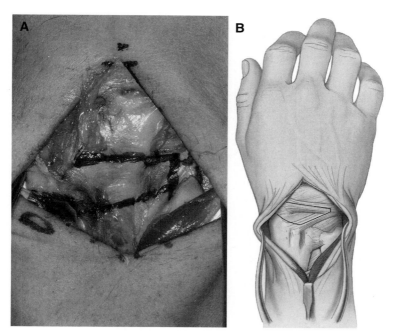

Fig. 9. (*A*) The ligament-sparing dorsal capsulotomy can be created using the radiotriquetral and scaphotriquetral ligaments, as shown in this clinical case (*lines drawn with marking pen*). To gain access to the radial aspect of the wrist, the capsule between the radius and scaphoid can be divided as well. (*B*) The ligament-sparing dorsal capsulotomy involves identification of the dorsal radiocarpal and dorsal intercarpal ligaments, followed by a fiber-splitting approach that bisects the ligaments (*lines*). To facilitate radial exposure, the radial origin of the dorsal radiocarpal ligament can be elevated toward the radial styloid and the capsule between the radius and scaphoid can be divided. (Copyright 2006 Mayo Clinics, reproduced with permission of the Mayo Foundation.)

Skin incision and subcutaneous tissue

There are many variations of the carpal tunnel approach; however, they are essentially all an extended open carpal tunnel release. One such incision follows the curve of the thenar muscles to the level of the wrist crease, and then extends proximally via a zigzag incision (Fig. 13A). The distal extent of the incision is Kaplan's cardinal line, and the proximal extent is determined by the surgeon. To minimize the chance of damage to the palmar cutaneous branch of the median nerve and its ulnar branches, the incision should be aligned between the long/ring finger web space [22] or 5 mm ulnar to the interthenar depression, which is the deepest point between the thenar and hypothenar eminences [23]. To avoid damaging the branches of the palmar cutaneous branch of the ulnar nerve, the palmar incision should not be sited any more ulnar than the longitudinal axis of the ring finger when extended [24]. At the level of the distal wrist crease, the incision should

be zigzagged, starting in an ulnar direction, into the distal forearm as needed. Care should be taken in designing the zigzag incision to avoid damaging the palmar cutaneous branch of the median nerve in the distal forearm [25] on the radial side, and the ulnar neurovascular bundle on the ulnar side. The superficial palmar fascia, with its longitudinal fibers, and the antebrachial fascia should then be incised in a longitudinal fashion (Fig. 13B).

Retinaculum

After identifying the median nerve proximally, which is radial and deep to the palmaris longus tendon, the flexor retinaculum is identified. The flexor retinaculum has thick transverse crisscross fibers, and is divided on the ulnar aspect of the carpal canal just radial to the hook of the hamate (Fig. 13C). The contents of the carpal canal can be looped in a Penrose drain and retracted radially or ulnarly to expose the volar wrist capsule and the pronator quadratus muscle (Fig. 13D).

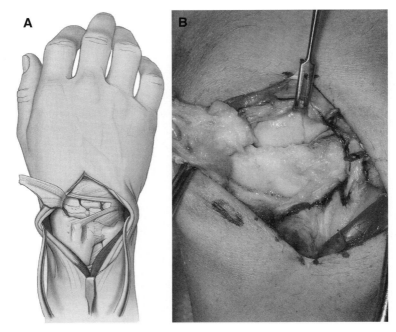

Fig. 10. (*A*) On completion of the dorsal capsulotomy, the scaphoid, lunate, and portions of the capitate and triquetrum are immediately visible. (Copyright 2006 Mayo Clinics, reproduced with permission of the Mayo Foundation.) (*B*) Appropriate retractions of the capsule and palmar flexion of the wrist will maximize the full exposure potential of this capsulotomy.

Capsule

Here again, the palmar wrist capsule contains important capsular ligaments [4–6]. To avoid potential postoperative problems associated with ulnar translation of the carpus, efforts should be made to minimize ligament disruption. This can be accomplished by leaving the long radiolunate ligament intact. This ligament tethers the triquetrum to the radius with the palmar lunotriquetral ligament [6]. Thus, the interligamentous sulcus or the space of Poirier is the first place to begin the capsulotomy using a fiber-splitting approach. If additional exposure is required on the radial side, a subperiosteal elevation of the radial origin of the radioscaphocapite ligament or the long radiolunate ligament (but preferably not both), can be performed continuing from the incision in the space of Poirier. Typically, this approach is used to repair the injured space of Poirer in perilunate fracture dislocations (Fig. 14).

Volar carpal exposure: modified Henry approach

The modified Henry or trans-flexor carpi radialis (FCR) approach is a popular approach for exposure of the volar surface of the distal radius. Appropriate capsulotomies from the origins of the radiocarpal ligaments could also provide access to the radiocarpal joint, proximal scaphoid, and lunate.

Skin and subcutaneous tissue

A longitudinal incision over the FCR tendon is carried proximally for 3 to 4 cm. Care must be taken not to cross the ulnar border of the FCR tendon, because the palmar cutaneous branch of the median nerve lies there.

Deeper dissection

The FCR tendon sheath is divided longitudinally to expose the FCR tendon. Retraction of the FCR tendon will reveal the floor the FCR tendon sheath. Another longitudinal incision is made through the floor of the FCR tendon sheath and the underlying connective tissue. On the radial side of the FCR tendon sheath, the radial artery and its venae comitantes can be visualized. Care must be taken to protect this vascular structure. The pronator quadratus muscle will be encountered. An incision is made along its distal margin. Retraction of the FCR tendon and radial artery radially will

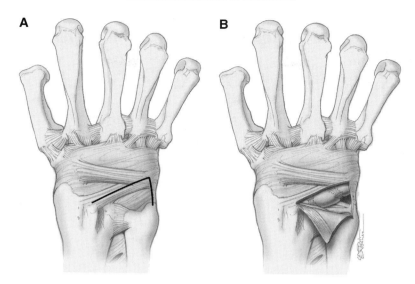

Fig. 11. (*A*) Ligament-sparing capsulotomy for exposure of the ulnocarpal joint; line shows incision path. Care should be taken during this procedure not to injure the triangular fibrocartilage complex. (*B*) Completion of the ulnocarpal capsulotomy showing adequate dorsal exposure of the triangular fibrocartilage complex, proximal surfaces of the lunate and triquetrum, and the lunotriquetral joint. (*A* and *B* copyright 2006 Mayo Clinics, reproduced with permission of the Mayo Foundation.)

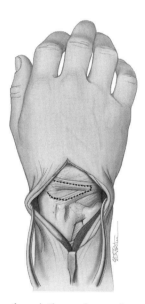

Fig. 12. After the wrist has undergone its surgical procedure, closure is performed anatomically. The capsulotomy is closed by nonabsorbable sutures. Because there is no complete transaction of the dorsal carpal ligaments, there is no need for high-strength repairs. The extensor tendons are replaced and the extensor retinaculum is closed, transposing the extensor pollicus longus dorsal to the retinaculum. (Copyright 2006 Mayo Clinics, reproduced with permission of the Mayo Foundation.)

expose the radial margin of the pronator quadratus muscle. An incision is made on the radial margin, leaving a 1 cm cuff of muscle on the radial side for later repair. The pronator quadratus muscle can now be elevated subperiosteally in a radial to ulnar direction to expose the volar surface of the distal radius and the volar radiocarpal wrist capsule. Self-retaining retractors can now be inserted into the wound, with the pronator quadratus muscle bulk on the ulnar side protecting the flexor tendons and median nerve, and the FCR tendon and radial artery on the radial side.

Volar exposure of the scaphoid: specific

The volar approach to the scaphoid was popularized by Russe after his description of scaphoid fracture nonunion repair [26–28]. This approach is primarily indicated for the open reduction and fixation of scaphoid waist or distal pole fractures. The advantages of this approach include preservation of the vascularity of the scaphoid by avoiding the dorsal distal blood supply, and an easier ability to correct apex dorsal angulations (humpback deformity) of scaphoid waist non-unions or malunions [29]; however, one problem with the approach is the potential of carpal instability as a result of the required

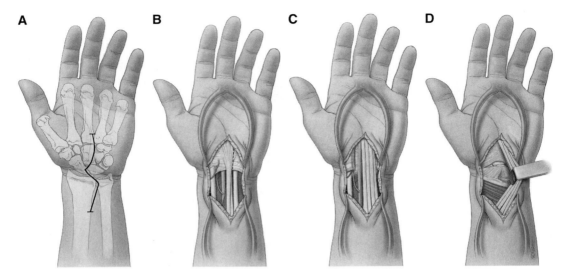

Fig. 13. (*A*) Design of the extended carpal tunnel skin incision for exposure of the volar carpus (*zigzag line*). Care must be taken in its location and design to preserve the palmar cutaneous branch of the median nerve and its ulnar branches, the palmar cutaneous branch of the ulnar nerve, and the ulnar neurovascular bundle. (*B*) Once through the skin and subcutaneous tissue, the superficial palmar fascia will be encountered in the hand and in the forearm, the thin antebrachial fascia. These fibers can be split or incised in a longitudinal manner until the transverse fibers of the flexor retinaculum are identified (*dashed lines*). (*C*) After incising the flexor retinaculum (dashed line), the retinacular flaps can be held open with self-retaining retractors to expose the contents of the carpal tunnel. (*D*) Gentle retraction of the flexor tendons and the median nerve will allow exposure of the volar capsule of the wrist joint. In cases of perilunate fracture dislocations, a transverse rent in the Space of Poirier can be identified, as illustrated here (*A–D* copyright 2006 Mayo Clinics, reproduced with permission of the Mayo Foundation.)

division of the radiocarpal ligaments (radioscaphocapitate and long radiolunate ligaments) [30].

Skin incision and subcutaneous tissue

A longitudinal incision, over the FCR tendon is carried proximally for 1.5 to 2 cm from scaphoid tuberosity. The distal incision angles toward and is in line with the thumb metacarpal (Fig. 15A). Care must be taken not to cross the ulnar border of the FCR because the palmar cutaneous branch of the median nerve lies there.

Deeper dissection

The FCR tendon sheath is then divided longitudinally, and the tendon is mobilized as far as the scaphoid tuberosity distally and retracted ulnarward. In the distal portion of the wound, it will be necessary to ligate and divide the superficial branch of the radial artery, which at times can be quite sizeable (Fig. 15B,C). The deep tendon sheath of the FCR tendon is divided longitudinally, together with the pericapsular fat underlying it. Division of the pericapsular fat will

reveal the palmar wrist capsule, which in this region contains the capsular ligaments of the radioscaphocapitate and the long radiolunate ligament (Fig. 15D). The long radiolunate and radioscaphocapitate ligaments are sharply divided (Fig. 15E), exposing the scaphoid waist (Fig. 15F).

Closure

The radioscaphocapitate and long radiolunate ligaments must be repaired stoutly with sutures if one is to avoid potential carpal stability problems [30].

Dorsal exposure of the schaphoid: specific

The dorsal approach to the scaphoid provides better access to the proximal scaphoid, and is indicated in the fixation of proximal scaphoid fractures. There is a concern with injury to the vascular supply of the scaphoid; however, recent reports have not shown a significant difference in the union rates when compared with the volar approach [31].

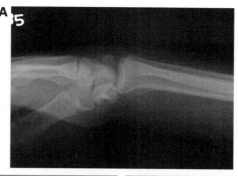

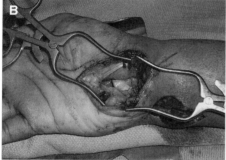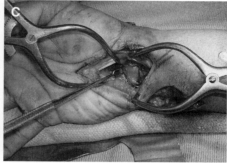

Fig. 14. (*A*) Perilunate fracture dislocation injury (Mayfield Stage IV) demonstrating lunate dislocation on lateral radiograph. (*B*) The lunate is seen lying in the carpal tunnel following an extended carpal tunnel exposure. The distal articular surface of the lunate is visualized. (*C*) The transverse rent in the space of Poirier following reduction of the lunate. Often a combined volar and dorsal approach is required. Once surgical reduction and repairs are completed, the space of Poirier should be repaired.

Skin incision

The dorsal approach to the scaphoid is performed through a transverse or longitudinal incision over the scapholunate interval and radiocarpal joint. A longitudinal incision is least likely to injure branches of the superficial radial nerve compared with a transverse incision, although it is less cosmetic.

Retinaculum

After skin flaps are elevated and the superficial branch of the radial nerve is identified and protected, the extensor retinaculum over the third dorsal compartment is opened and the extensor policis longus (EPL) tendon is retracted radially. The septum between the third and fourth compartments is opened as described in the dorsal approach to the carpus, and the extensor tendons are retracted ulnarward.

Capsule

Radial to the insertion of the dorsal radiocarpal ligament, there are no true ligamentous structures; only capsule is present. The capsule can be opened between the radius and scaphoid radial to the border of the dorsal radiocarpal ligament. If further exposure is necessary, the ligament can be divided longitudinally along its fibers, creating a distally based flap.

Exposure

The entire proximal two thirds of the scaphoid, the radial styloid, and the scaphoid fossa in the distal radius can be exposed.

Closure

The capsule is easily closed with sutures irrespective of the type of capsulotomy used. The EPL tendon is transposed dorsal to the repaired retinaculum.

Approach to distal radioulnar joint: specific

The distal radioulnar joint can be exposed dorsally through a 4 cm longitudinal skin incision made between the fifth and sixth extensor

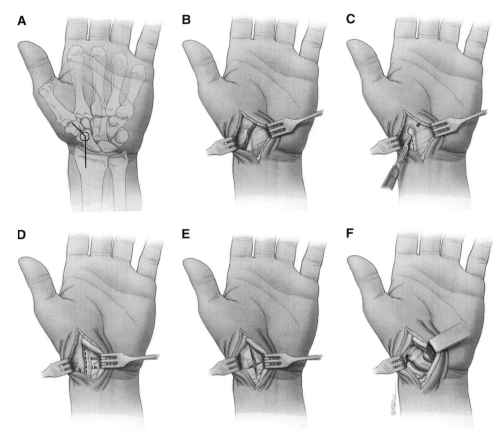

Fig. 15. (*A*) Skin incision for volar exposure of the scaphoid (*angled line*) is centered around the scaphoid tuberosity (*circle*). (*B*) The superficial branch of the radial artery and its venae comitantes will cross the incision and will require division. (*C*) The superficial surface of the flexor carpi radialis tendon sheath is incised longitudinally (*dashed line*) to allow release of the tendon. (*D*) The flexor carpi radialis tendon is retracted to allow exposure of the deep volar surface of the tendon sheath. The volar sheath of the flexor carpi radialis is intimately associated with the radioscaphocapitate (*RSC*) and long radiolunate ligaments (*LRL*), which need to be divided to expose the scaphoid waist. A longitudinal incision (*dotted line*) is made in the floor of the sheath, dividing the RSC and LRL. (*E*) The long radiolunate and the radioscaphocapitate ligament should be sharply incised to allow later repair. Care should be taken not to injure the underlying cartilage of the scaphoid. (*F*) Complete exposure of the volar surface of the scaphoid is achieved with appropriate retraction. (*A–F* copyright 2006 Mayo Clinics, reproduced with permission of the Mayo Foundation.)

compartments, extending proximally from the level of the ulnar styloid [32]. The fifth compartment lies right over the distal radioulnar joint. The retinaculum over the fifth compartment should be opened and the extensor digiti minimi tendon should be retracted. An L-shaped ulnar based capsular flap is created by incising the dorsal capsule of the distal radioulnar joint along the radial attachment, leaving a small rim of capsule for subsequent repair. The capsulotomy extends distally to the level of the dorsal radioulnar ligament, which appears as a distinct thickening of the capsule as the sigmoid notch is approached. The capsulotomy extends ulnarly along the proximal edge of the dorsal radioulnar ligament until the sixth compartment is reached.

This exposure will allow unencumbered visualization of the distal radioulnar joint, and by rotating the forearm, the entire surface of the ulnar head articulating with the sigmoid notch of the radius can be visualized. By leaving the dorsal radioulnar ligament, the stability of the joint is not compromised. Direct repair of the capsulotomy is easily completed along the distal and radial extents.

Summary

The current surgical approaches to the carpus and the distal radioulnar joint are presented in this article. Although there are multiple modifications of these exposures that continue to evolve, the basics principles of the exposures are important to remember. As much as possible, ligament-sparing approaches should be used to minimize potential problems related to postoperative carpal instability and scarring, which may limit motion. Familiarity with these approaches, and more important, the anatomy of the carpus and surrounding tissues, will allow the surgeon to access virtually any part of the wrist.

References

[1] Nakamura A, Yamada T, Goto A, et al. Somatosensory homunculus as drawn by MEG. Neuroimage 1998;7:377–86.

[2] Nelson AW. The painful neuroma: the regenerating axon verus the epineural sheath. J Surg Res 1977;23: 215–21.

[3] Hazari A, Elliot D. Treatment of end-neuromas, neuromas-in-continuity and scarred nerves of the digits by proximal relocation. J Hand Surg [Br] 2004;29:338–50.

[4] Berger RA. The anatomy of the ligaments of the wrist and distal radioulnar joints. Clin Orthop Relat Res 2001;32–40.

[5] Berger RA. The ligaments of the wrist. A current overview of anatomy with considerations of their potential functions. Hand Clin 1997;13:63–82.

[6] Berger RA. Ligament anatomy. In: Cooney WP, Linscheid RL, Dobyns JH, editors. The wrist: diagnosis and operative treatment, vol. 1. St Louis (MO): Mosby; 1998. p. 73–105.

[7] Berger RA, Bishop AT, Bettinger PC. New dorsal capsulotomy for the surgical exposure of the wrist. Ann Plast Surg 1995;35:54–9.

[8] Millender LH, Nalebuff EA. Arthrodesis of the rheumatoid wrist. An evaluation of sixty patients and a description of a different surgical technique. J Bone Joint Surg Am 1973;55:1026–34.

[9] Potts H, Noble J. Surgical approaches to the dorsum of the wrist: brief report. J Bone Joint Surg Br 1988; 70:328–9.

[10] Auerbach DM, Collins ED, Kunkle KL, et al. The radial sensory nerve. An anatomic study. Clin Orthop Relat Res 1994;241–9.

[11] Abrams RA, Brown RA, Botte MJ. The superficial branch of the radial nerve: an anatomic study with surgical implications. J Hand Surg [Am] 1992;17: 1037–41.

[12] Bas H, Kleinert JM. Anatomic variations in sensory innervation of the hand and digits. J Hand Surg [Am] 1999;24:1171–84.

[13] Grossman JA, Yen L, Rapaport D. The dorsal cutaneous branch of the ulnar nerve. An anatomic clarification with six case reports. Chir Main 1998;17: 154–8.

[14] Ikiz ZA, Ucerler H. Anatomic characteristics and clinical importance of the superficial branch of the radial nerve. Surg Radiol Anat 2004;26: 453–8.

[15] Palmer AK, Skahen JR, Werner FW, et al. The extensor retinaculum of the wrist: an anatomical and biomechanical study. J Hand Surg [Br] 1985;10: 11–6.

[16] Dellon AL. Partial dorsal wrist denervation: resection of the distal posterior interosseous nerve. J Hand Surg [Am] 1985;10:527–33.

[17] Weinstein LP, Berger RA. Analgesic benefit, functional outcome, and patient satisfaction after partial wrist denervation. J Hand Surg [Am] 2002;27:833–9.

[18] Mitsuyasu H, Patterson RM, Shah MA, et al. The role of the dorsal intercarpal ligament in dynamic and static scapholunate instability. J Hand Surg [Am] 2004;29:279–88.

[19] Mayfield JK. Mechanism of carpal injuries. Clin Orthop Relat Res 1980;45–54.

[20] Mayfield JK, Johnson RP, Kilcoyne RK. Carpal dislocations: pathomechanics and progressive perilunar instability. J Hand Surg [Am] 1980;5: 226–41.

[21] Mayfield JK. Patterns of injury to carpal ligaments. A spectrum. Clin Orthop Relat Res 1984; 36–42.

[22] Ruch DS, Marr A, Holden M, et al. Innervation density of the base of the palm. J Hand Surg [Am] 1999;24:392–7.

[23] Watchmaker GP, Weber D, Mackinnon SE. Avoidance of transection of the palmar cutaneous branch of the median nerve in carpal tunnel release. J Hand Surg [Am] 1996;21:644–50.

[24] Martin CH, Seiler JG 3rd, Lesesne JS. The cutaneous innervation of the palm: an anatomic study of the ulnar and median nerves. J Hand Surg [Am] 1996;21:634–8.

[25] Matloub HS, Yan JG, Mink Van Der Molen AB, et al. The detailed anatomy of the palmar cutaneous nerves and its clinical implications. J Hand Surg [Br] 1998;23:373–9.

[26] Russe O. Experience and results in filling up of the substantia spongiosa in old fractures and pseudarthrosis of the scaphoid bone of the hand. Wiederherstellungschir Traumatol 1954;II:175–84 [in German].

[27] Russe O. Follow-up study results of 22 cases of operated old fractures and pseudarthroses of the scaphoid bone of the hand. Z Orthop Ihre Grenzgeb 1960; 93:5–14 [in German].

[28] Russe O. A Proven surgical technique in pseudarthrosis of the scaphoid bone of the hand. Klin Med Osterr Z Wiss Prakt Med 1964;19:100–1 [in German].

[29] Fernandez DL. A technique for anterior wedge-shaped grafts for scaphoid nonunions with carpal instability. J Hand Surg [Am] 1984;9:733–7.

[30] Garcia-Elias M, Vall A, Salo JM, et al. Carpal alignment after different surgical approaches to the scaphoid: a comparative study. J Hand Surg [Am] 1988;13:604–12.

[31] Polsky MB, Kozin SH, Porter ST, et al. Scaphoid fractures: dorsal versus volar approach. Orthopedics 2002;25:817–9.

[32] Adams BD, Berger RA. An anatomic reconstruction of the distal radioulnar ligaments for posttraumatic distal radioulnar joint instability. J Hand Surg [Am] 2002;27:243–51.

ELSEVIER
SAUNDERS

Hand Clin 22 (2006) 435–446

HAND
CLINICS

Lesions and Tumors of the Carpus

Christopher L. Forthman, MD[a],*, Keith A. Segalman, MD[b]

[a]Curtis National Hand Center, Union Memorial Hospital, 3333 North Calvert Street, 2nd Floor,
Baltimore, MD 21218, USA
[b]Department of Orthopaedic Surgery, Johns Hopkins School of Medicine, 601 North Caroline Street,
Baltimore, MD 21287-0765, USA

Wrist pain is one of the most common complaints seen by a hand or orthopedic surgeon. The proximate cause is often obvious, but a cursory examination may allow the clinician to miss significant underyling pathology (Fig. 1). A careful, thorough examination is warranted, even when the diagnosis seems apparent. The hand surgeon should be familiar with neoplasms that may affect the carpus, in order to accurately diagnose and treat patients who have wrist pain.

Evaluating a carpal lesion

The differential diagnosis for lesions and tumors within the carpus is broad. The distinguishing clinical and radiographic features of these entities seen elsewhere in the body are often absent in the wrist, owing to the diminutive size of the carpal bones. For example, pathologic fracture may occur through a carpal tumor without the antecedent pain and classic osteolytic or permeative radiographic appearance seen in a long bone. On the other hand, small lesions that are usually asymptomatic elsewhere in the body may cause significant discomfort in the wrist. A half-centimeter size intraosseous lesion will compromise a relatively large portion of the osseous architecture of a carpal bone; enough disruption to elicit pain. Nevertheless, not all lesions and tumors of the carpus are symptomatic, and they may even distract the surgeon and patient from the true diagnosis. The hand surgeon has the challenging task of not only identifying and differentiating these lesions and tumors, but also of determining which radiographic findings are incidental.

The history and physical examination should correlate with the radiographic appearance and location of the lesion. The authors have found that point tenderness over the affected carpal bone is the most sensitive indicator that a lesion is clinically significant. The degree of pain often corresponds with the metabolic activity of the lesion, as indicated by changes in the osseous architecture. Plain radiographs and CT should be examined for subtle indicators of bone turnover such as lytic or sclerotic areas. More dramatic findings such as cortical erosion or pathologic fracture are less commonly present, but suggest the possibility of a neoplasm. The authors have found a bone scan to be useful to confirm the presence of a true tumor (eg, osteoid osteoma) or other highly metabolically active processes (eg, osteomyelitis) (Fig. 2).

MRI may be obtained to further evaluate the painful wrist. The authors typically request an MRI to exclude other carpal pathology, and to evaluate the internal soft tissue architecture of the lesion. An MRI is particularly valuable in patients who have wrist pain but a physical examination that is inconsistent with the radiographically identified carpal lesion. In these cases, the MRI will commonly reveal other pathology (eg, triangular fibrocartilage complex [TFCC] tear) more compatible with the patient's symptoms. The MRI also defines the soft tissue components of the lesion itself. T1 images show fine anatomic

---

* Corresponding author. Greater Chesapeake Hand Specialists, 1400 Front Street, Suite 100, Lutherville, MD 21093.
 E-mail address: clforthman@yahoo.com (C.L. Forthman).

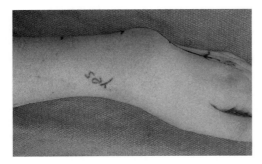

Fig. 1. Giant cell tumor of the carpus misdiagnosed as a dorsal wrist ganglion.

detail and have high signal intensity for fat (as well as gadolinium, proteinaceous fluid, methemoblobin/blood, and melanin). T2 fat-suppressed and short tau inversion recovery (STIR) sequences are water-sensitive, and will identify fluid-filled cysts as well as the edema that accompanies injury (eg, ligament tears, pathologic fractures), infection, or infiltrating tumors. Careful review of the MRI is often the final step necessary for planning the definitive surgery for most lesions and tumors of the carpus.

Lesions that are especially destructive or that infiltrate the soft tissues may need further workup. The surgeon should exclude inflammatory processes such as rheumatoid arthritis, gout, and infection, all of which are more common than a true aggressive tumor or lesion of the carpus (Fig. 3). The wrist is aspirated for infection, serology is sent for autoimmune synovitis, anti-inflammatory drugs are prescribed for an inflammatory

arthropathy, and so on. If a true aggressive or malignant lesion is suspected, the authors obtain routine laboratory studies, a chest radiograph, a CT scan of the chest and abdomen, and an incisional biopsy. At the surgeon's discretion, the biopsy may be performed before the other studies to avoid unnecessary workup. The biopsy is planned so that it can be incorporated into an extensile exposure for excision of the tumor en bloc. The sections that follow provide details to help the hand surgeon identify and treat specific lesions and tumors of the carpus.

Intraosseous ganglion

Epidemiology

The most common carpal lesion is the intraosseous ganglion (IOG). Also known as a subchondral bone cyst, the IOG is a benign, mucin-filled, cystlike lesion that arises within the subchondral medullary bone. IOGs are regularly seen on wrist radiographs obtained to evaluate wrist pain or other problems. In a radiographic study of 280 cadaveric wrists, Schrank and colleagues [1] identified an overall 9.6% incidence of carpal ganglion cysts. In patients who have dorsal wrist ganglions, the prevalence of IOGs is reported to be almost 50% [2]. Like soft tissue ganglia, IOGs occur adjacent to synovial lined joint structures and are usually filled with a gelatinous material.

Intraosseous ganglia are identified most often in middle-aged patients. Radiographs show an eccentric intraosseous radiolucent lesion with a sclerotic sharp margin located close to the

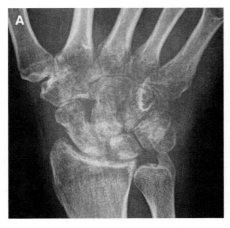

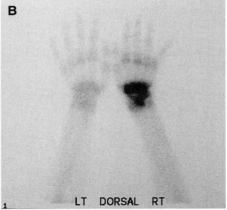

Fig. 2. Osteomyelitis. (*A*) Plain radiographs demonstrate diffuse sclerotic and lytic changes in the carpus. (*B*) Bone scan confirms an active inflammatory, infectious, or neoplastic process.

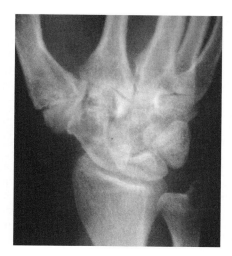

Fig. 3. Radiographs demonstrate a destructive lesion involving the scaphoid and trapezoid. Close inspection reveals a silicone thumb carpometacarpal implant (silicone synovitis).

carpal bone surface. Intraosseous ganglia are well-circumscribed and generally do not have an identifiable macroscopic penetration of the cortex. Rarely, cortical disruption can be seen in the region of a nearby ligament attachment site; however, the penetration is distant from the subchondral bone of the joint, and the joint remains covered with hyaline cartilage [1,3,4]. Any carpal bone may be affected, but the lunate, capitate, and scaphoid are the most frequent [1,2,5–8]. Lesions may occur in multiple carpal bones, and may be bilateral [3,9,10].

Pathogenesis

The pathogenesis of the IOG is controversial. In some cases the lesion arises adjacent to an area of repeated osseous microtrauma. A synovial leak may occur with focal avascular necrosis and subsequent ganglion formation (Fig. 4) [11]. In the cadaveric examinations performed by Schrank and colleagues [1], the majority of intraosseous carpal ganglions(89.5%) were in close proximity to the insertion of the capsule, the scapholunate, or the lunatotriquetral ligament. The study authors concluded that inclusions of fluid because of carpal ligament pathology is probably the process that initiates the formation of the ganglia [1]. The high prevalence of intraosseous ganglia in patients who have dorsal wrist ganglia supports this theory [2].

Schajowicz and colleagues [11] categorized IOGs as those that follow the penetration of juxtaosseous material into bone, "penetrating type," and those which are primarily intraosseous, "idiopathic type." Perhaps the later type may arise from primary intramedullary metaplasia [12]. Regardless of the etiology, the ganglion wall is composed of fibrous, collagenous fibers with mucoid-degeneration and no clear epithelial or synovial cell lining. The surrounding bone is focally sclerotic and, by microscopic examination, has components of both necrotic and revascularized osseous elements [1,11].

The IOG should be differentiated from a degenerative osteoarthritic cyst. Unlike the fully circumscribed IOG, degenerative cysts often connect with the joint space via macroscopic crevices and erosions [13]. Histologically, arthritic cysts

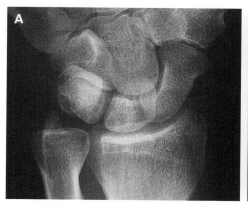
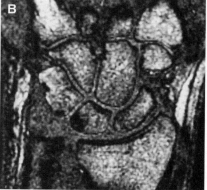

Fig. 4. Ulnocarpal impaction. (*A*) Plain radiographs show ulnar positive variance and subtle lytic lesions in the lunate and triquetrum. (*B*) MRI confirms focal replacement of the normal fatty marrow elements. These changes may be early in the process of ganglion (cyst) formation.

typically have a wall lined by a flat epithelium with a synovial covering [13]. Additionally, degenerative cysts are often accompanied by nearby arthritic changes such as subchondral sclerosis, osteophytes, and narrowing of the joint space. On direct inspection, eroded hyaline cartilage adjacent to the cystic lesion identifies the cyst as degenerative rather than as an IOG.

Clinical presentation

IOG may cause symptoms localized to the affected bone, and should be considered in the setting of pain without another clinical explanation. A negative bone scan does not exclude a symptomatic ganglion cyst or the need for surgical treatment. Nevertheless, IOGs are often asymptomatic, and pain should not be attributed to an IOG without excluding the possibility of another diagnosis (eg, osteoid osteoma) or other carpal pathology.

Axial imaging of the IOG demonstrates key diagnostic features. CT shows a well-circumscribed and purely lytic lesion, whereas MRI reveals the contents as a homogenous water equivalent signal (Fig. 5). If the internal architecture is more complex, then a different diagnosis such as osteoid osteoma or enchondroma should be strongly considered. MRI also allows evaluation for related adjacent ligament pathology or unrelated pain generators involving the ligamentous structures and cartilage surfaces.

Treatment

Symptomatic IOGs are successfully treated with curettage and bone grafting [3–5,7,10]. The authors make a generous window to completely evacuate the ganglion contents and, more importantly, the ganglion wall. A thorough curettage helps ensure that the lesion will not recur, even if the final pathology returns one of the neoplastic lesions described below. The cavity is conveniently packed with cancellous bone from the adjacent distal radius (Fig. 6). Although there is no conclusive evidence that bone grafting is required, the authors prefer to do so. Grafting restores the native architecture of the bone, and may expedite healing and pain relief postoperatively. Allograft bone or bone substitutes may also be used.

Benign bone tumors

Primary bone tumors of the carpus are rare [14]. The two most common lesions, osteoid osteoma and enchondroma, may be easily misdiagnosed as IOG. Enchondromas may cause pathologic fractures, especially of the scaphoid, just as they do in the phalanges. The giant cell tumor, although more often originating from the distal radius instead of the carpus, routinely causes carpal destruction. Other benign bone tumors, including osteochondroma, chrondroblastoma, chondromyxoid fibroma, hemangioma, aneurysmal bone cyst, and osteoblastoma, are described in case reports.

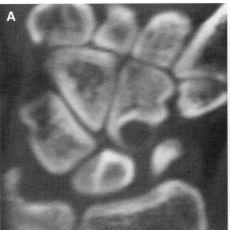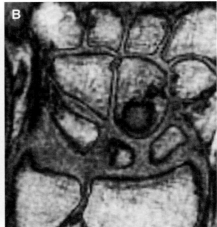

Fig. 5. Imaging an intraosseous ganglion of the capitate. (*A*) CT clarifies the sclerotic cortical rim that surrounds an IOG. (*B*) MRI illustrates the homogenous internal architecture expected of a ganglion.

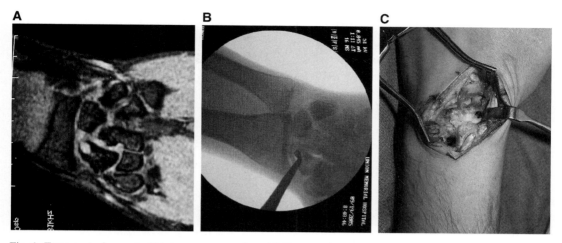

Fig. 6. Treatment of a scaphoid intraosseous ganglion. (*A*) Preoperative cross-sectional imaging precisely localizes the location of the lesion. (*B*) Intraoperative biplanar fluoroscopy facilitates precision curettage. (*C*) Graft is taken from the distal radius to reconstitute the bone of the proximal pole.

Osteoid osteoma

An osteoid osteoma is a benign osteoblastic tumor typically found in the long bones of persons between the ages of 10 and 30. It is composed of a central core of osteoid and bony trabeculae surrounded by highly vascular fibrous connective tissue. Grossly, the tumor is well-circumscribed, with a reddish-brown nidus.

Osteoid osteomas cause a constant focal pain at the site of the tumor. Pain is worse at night, and is dramatically relieved with small doses of aspirin or other salicylates. Although rare in the carpus, the osteoid osteoma must be considered in the differential diagnosis of wrist pain in adolescents or young adults [15,16]. The usual sign is point tenderness over the involved bone. A case of carpal tunnel syndrome has been attributed to an osteoid osteoma causing the contour of the capitate to project volarly into carpal canal [17].

Osteoid osteomas may be found anywhere in the carpus, but most lesions have been reported in the scaphoid, hamate, and capitate [16,18,19]. Classically, radiographs show a discrete central nidus of bone surrounded by an area of lucency enclosed within a dense ring of sclerosis; a target-shaped lesion. Within the diminutive bones of the hand and wrist, the tumor may appear purely osteolytic, similar to an IOG. Other atypical radiographic features may also be present, including subtle changes in bone density and cortical irregularities or hypertrophy. Plain radiographs may even be normal [20]. A bone scan shows very high technetium Tc 99m diphosphonate uptake. CT reliably identifies the bony nidus at the core of the tumor [16]. Roentgenographically distinct multiple nidi have been reported in the scaphoid and capitate [21].

An osteoid osteoma is never an incidental finding; pain is universal. Nonetheless, the tumor may regress spontaneously, so a period of aspirin therapy may be considered. In the wrist, lesions are surgically accessible, so all reports in the literature involve operative management. Resection of the nidus is curative [19,20,22] and recurrence is rare [16,23]. The authors pack the defect with local cancellous bone graft, although removing the lesion is clearly the most important factor in pain relief [22]. A recent study [24] demonstrated successful treatment of osteoid osteomas of the upper extremity using radiofrequency ablation; however, this technique is not currently recommended for the carpal bones because of the proximity of neurovascular structures.

Enchondroma

A chondroma is a benign cartilaginous neoplasm of bone. Usually the tumor arises within the medullary cavity of a tubular bone and is known as an enchondroma. A chondroma may also originate on the surface of bone—a juxtacortical or periosteal chondroma. The tumor is composed of mineralized or unmineralized hyaline cartilage, and appears pearly gray on gross inspection.

The enchondroma is the most common primary bone tumor in the hand, and has a particular predilection for the proximal phalanges of young adults. Less frequently, enchondromas of the hand occur in the metacarpal, followed by the middle phalanx, and lastly the carpus [25]. Takigawa [26] reviewed 110 cases of chondromas in the hand, and only identified two in the carpus, one scaphoid and one lunate. Similarly, as a proportion of all carpal lesions, enchondromas are uncommon. Of 86 carpal bone lesions treated by Emecheta and colleagues [27], only three were enchondromas.

Most carpal enchondromas occur in the scaphoid, and most are usually minimally symptomatic until a pathologic fracture occurs [26–31]. Takka and Poyraz [31] reviewed eight cases of scaphoid enchondroma in the literature, five of which presented with a pathologic fracture. In their case, an 11-year-old boy had mild pain but no fracture. Periosteal chondromas may cause mechanical or compressive symptoms, including carpal tunnel syndrome [32]. Malignant change is very rare in solitary chondromas, and it has not been reported in the carpus.

Enchondromas replace normal medullary bone, creating radiographically well-defined margins. In the hand, enchondromas may be quite expansive, commonly causing endosteal scalloping and significant cortical thinning. Chondral calcification occurs throughout the lesion and appears as rings and arcs on plain radiograph; a "stippled" appearance. CT clarifies this punctate matrix mineralization, distinguishing this lesion from an intraosseous ganglion, osteoid osteoma, or other process. CT is also useful for assessing the integrity of the cortex and the configuration of pathologic fractures.

Carpal enchondromas are treated more aggressively than those in the proximal phalanx, owing to the frequency of the tumor in the scaphoid and the risk of a pathologic fracture. Most carpal cases are treated with curettage and grafting of the lesion with autograft from the distal radius or iliac crest. Corticocancellous graft may sometimes by necessary to restore the osseous architecture of the scaphoid [27]. If the vascularity of the scaphoid is compromised by extensive curettage, a vascularized 1,2 intracompartmental supraretinacular artery graft may be used [28]. Notably, the osteolysis, sclerosis, and dystrophic calcification associated with a cystic scaphoid nonunion may be difficult to differentiate from the architecture of a pathologic scaphoid fracture caused by an enchondroma. The diagnosis is facilitated by MRI, which shows the nonmineralized portion of the enchondroma.

Giant cell tumor

A giant cell tumor (GCT) is a benign but locally aggressive tumor that should be considered in the differential diagnosis of any osteolytic bone lesion. The GCT is composed of multinucleated giant cells within a sea of homogenous stromal cells. Notably, giant cells may be present in other lesions found in the carpus, including aneurysmal bone cysts, chondroblastomas, chondromyxoid fibromas, the bone lesions of hyperparathyroidism, and giant cell-containing osteosarcomas.

GCTs are most common in skeletally mature young adults. The tumors generally present with slowly progressive pain, and sometimes a soft tissue mass. Radiographs demonstrate a well-defined radiolucency in the epiphyseal region of a long bone. The tumor obliterates the medullary cavity, and often expands through the adjacent cortex. The distal radius is the third most common site for GCTs and, not infrequently these lesions are aggressive enough to involve the nearby carpus.

GCTs may also arise primarily from a carpal bone. In a review of previously published series, Averill and colleagues [33] found 4 of 1200 GCTs originating in the carpus. Overall, 2% of GCTs occur in the bones of the hand, and 18% percent of GCTs in the hand are multicentric. Averill and colleagues [33] recommend a bone scan to look for additional foci when a GCT in the hand is identified. In their series of 28 GCTs of the hand, the authors report one case in the carpus—a multicentric tumor of the hamate and trapezoid [33].

Patients who have GCTs of the carpus complain of dorsal wrist swelling, pain, and limited motion. Symptoms may mimic other diseases such as basal joint arthritis [34]. Unlike the radiographic appearance of GCTs elsewhere, GCTs of the carpus typically manifest as a radiolucency without expansion of the bone [33–38]. Differentiation from other carpal lesions such as an intraosseous ganglion is difficult. FitzPatrick and Bullough [38] reported a case of the lunate that radiographically appeared to be Kienböck's disease.

GCTs localized to a carpal bone are best treated by en bloc excision of the affected bone. Curettage alone has a 100% recurrence rate, and curettage with adjuvant (eg, liquid nitrogen) has not been proven more effective. Lane and colleagues [35] reported cases of GCTs in the lunate and capitate that recurred after curettage and grafting. Likewise, a GCT of the capitate recurred after curettage and grafting by Howard and

Lassen [36]. All three of these cases resolved after total or near total excision of the carpal bone. In cases treated primarily with excision of the affected bone, there have been no reported recurrences [37,38].

GCTs of the carpus have the potential to infiltrate the adjacent tissues, similar to GCTs of the distal radius. Weiner and Leeson [34] reported a case of a GCT of the trapezium that invaded into the trapezoid and thenar musculature. The authors have seen a very aggressive GCT destroy the entire proximal carpal row, and infiltrate volarly and dorsally into the adjacent soft tissues (Fig. 7). Wide excision of expansive tumors is necessary, because the most important factor governing the rate of local recurrence is the margin at the time of the surgical procedure. The entire carpus and some of the distal radius may need to be removed. Reconstruction may require wrist fusion, possibly using a free vascularized fibula graft as described in the literature for distal radius GCTs [39–43].

Other benign bone tumors

The carpal bones develop as expanding chondral centers of ossification, and can potentially be home to any musculoskeletal neoplasm that occurs in cartilage or bone. Chondroblastoma [44] and chondrommyxoid fibroma [45] are rare chondral lesions in the carpus. Osteoblastoma, the larger counterpart of the osteoid osteoma, is an uncommon bone producing carpal tumor [46,47]. The osteochondroma also may originate in the carpus and cause tendon irritation and other mechanical symptoms [48,49]. Finally,

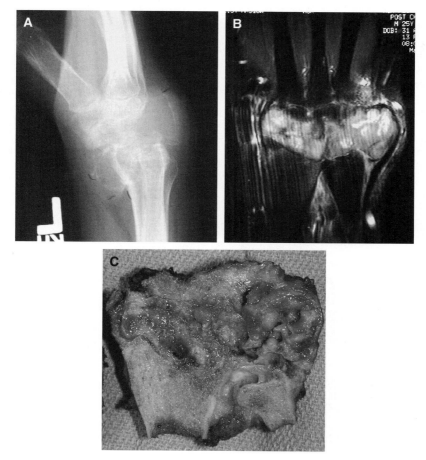

Fig. 7. Giant cell tumor of the wrist. (*A*) Lateral radiograph shows the expansive osteolytic appearance characteristic of GCTs about the wrist. (*B*) MRI demonstrates infiltration of the tumor into the adjacent soft tissues. (*C*) Bivalved specimen reveals preservation of the distal radius and obliteration of the carpus, suggesting a carpal origin for the tumor.

benign bone tumors may contain an aneurysmal bone cyst (ABC), or an ABC may arise de novo in the carpus [50,51]. In each case, curettage and grafting is an acceptable preliminary surgical treatment, because the diagnosis is often not made until pathologic examination.

Intra-articular tumors

Intra-articular tumors of the wrist should be considered as a possible cause of generalized wrist swelling, pain, and stiffness. Plain radiographs often do not provide many clues to the underlying diagnosis. CT or MRI will show the extent of the disease, but the hand surgeon may still confuse the tumor with an inflammatory process such as rheumatoid arthritis or gout (Fig. 8). The features of the axial images must be reviewed carefully, just as the surgeon would critically examine any abnormal tissue seen intraoperatively.

Pigmented villonodular synovitis

Pigmented villonodular synovitis (PVNS) is a benign tumor characterized by synovial hyperplasia and a proliferation of multinucleated giant cells. Hemosiderin is found within the cells and surrounding tissues, creating a pigmented tan or brownish-yellow appearance to the lesions. Grossly, PVNS occurs in two forms, nodular and diffuse. Both forms may occur in young to middle-aged adults around the synovial sites of the hand.

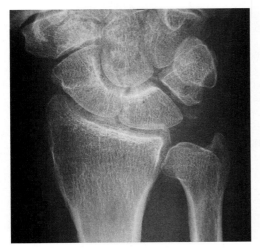

Fig. 8. Plain radiographs demonstrate chondrocalcinosis about the ulnocarpal joint in a patient with pseudogout.

PVNS is usually encountered by hand surgeons in its nodular form, a localized nodular tenosynovitis, also known as giant cell tumor of the tendon sheath. These circumscribed lesions are most common about the palmar surfaces of the fingers, and may erode into the underlying bone [52]. The diffuse form of the disease occurs in the wrist and, although much less common [53,54], it has the same ability to invade local tissues [55–59].

PVNS of the wrist causes a mildly painful swollen joint. Aspiration yields dark-brown, hemorrhagic synovial fluid that suggests the diagnosis. Plain radiographs show carpal bone erosions or cysts, but intralesional calcifications are uncommon. As a result, the true extent of the mass is not readily apparent on radiographs, and the diagnosis is often delayed. Carpintero [55] and colleagues reported a case initially misdiagnosed as an intraosseous ganglion.

Cross-sectional imaging reveals the diagnosis by demonstrating the intra-articular soft tissue mass responsible for the effusion and carpal bone findings. On CT examination the mass is hyperdense secondary to frequent hemorrhage and blood breakdown products. On MRI the mass may demonstrate the full spectrum of signal intensity, depending on the region of the tumor. Acute bleeding will have high signal intensity on T2-weighted images, whereas hemosiderin has low signal intensity on T1 and T2 sequences.

Overall, MRI allows preoperative planning for resection of the soft tissue mass, whereas CT examination facilitates management of changes in the bony architecture.

PVNS of the wrist is treated by a complete synovectomy, including dorsal and volar incisions as needed. Acute carpal tunnel syndrome [60] or more chronic median neuropathy [55] may need to be addressed concurrently. It is worthwhile in joints with minimal destruction to attempt curettage and bone grafting of carpal cysts. If tumor remains, the graft may resorb and the disease may progress, necessitating limited or total wrist arthrodesis for pain relief [55].

Synovial chondromatosis

Synovial chondromatosis is a metaplastic process of periarticular synovium, resulting in the formation of hyaline cartilage bodies. The cartilage bodies are usually gray-white in color, several millimeters in size, and found imbedded within the proliferative synovial membrane or free within the intra-articular space. The result is a painful, swollen joint, typically in a young to middle-aged adult—similar to PVNS. Loose bodies may cause catching or locking and ultimately arthritis from articular wear.

Synovial chondromatosis about the carpus is rare, but it must be considered in the differential of a painful, swollen, and stiff wrist. Loonen and Schuurman [61] recently reviewed the literature and identified 24 cases of synovial chondromatosis of the wrist, in addition to one of their own. Both the radiocarpal and distal radioulnar joints may be affected [62,63].

Plain radiographs often show characteristic calcified cartilaginous nodules, facilitating differentiation from PVNS and other synovial diseases. CT scan will further delineate calcified bodies that are not visible on plain radiograph. Both CT and MRI reveal the true extent of the disease, and may detect the early changes of secondary arthritis that inevitably occur. Synovial chondromatosis with secondary arthritic changes should not be confused with the more common clinical scenario of primary osteoarthritis with osteophytes, subchondral sclerosis, and loose osteochondral fragments.

The treatment of synovial chondromatosis involves synovectomy and removal of loose bodies. Symptoms improve with surgery, and few recurrences have been reported. Bone erosions and cysts are uncommon compared with PVNS, but secondary arthritic changes may need to be addressed, particularly if disease recurs [61].

Malignant bone tumors

Malignant bone tumors of the carpus are extraordinarily uncommon. Osteosarcoma, the most common malignant bone tumor, has only been reported in the carpus twice in the English literature [64,65]. Bickerstaff and colleagues [65] describe a 66-year-old female who had osteosarcoma of the trapezium, causing symptoms similar to arthritis of the thumb carpometacarpal joint. Marcuzzi and colleagues [64] tell of an osteosarcoma of the scaphoid mistaken for a benign lesion and treated with curettage and bone grafting.

Chondrosarcoma is the most common malignant bone tumor of the hand, but it too has only been reported twice in the carpus [66,67]. Of 30 cases in the hands and feet, Dahlin and colleagues [66] identified one case in the trapezoid. Granberry and Brylan [67] encountered a case in the trapezium initially treated as carpometacarpal arthritis of the thumb. Of interest, all four cases of

these malignant bone tumors occurred near the base of the thumb, and a malignant process was not suspected. These cases re-emphasize the need for the hand surgeon to maintain a high level of vigilance when reviewing any radiographic studies, even when the diagnosis seems straightforward.

Metastatic tumors

Metastatic disease in the hand is also very rare, but it is occasionally the first sign of an underlying cancer. In a review of world literature, Kerin [68] found that only about 0.1% of primary tumors metastasize to the hand. In almost 20% of these tumors, the lesion in the hand was the first indication of a primary tumor elsewhere. The most common source was bronchial carcinoma, and the terminal phalanges were the typical site of metastatic disease. Metastatic lesions were less frequently seen in the other phalanges and the metacarpals; one case occurred in the carpus.

The few reports of metastases to the carpus are typically from bronchial carcinoma, although metastases from other tumors such as prostate, breast, larynx, stomach, and bone sarcoma have been described [8,68–79]. Ioia and colleagues [77] reported a case of metastatic bronchial carcinoma to the scaphoid presenting with wrist pain, swelling, and tenderness. The radiographic lesion was initially misdiagnosed as an old scaphoid fracture, reminding the hand surgeon to remain cautious when evaluating any lesion of the wrist.

Patients who have metastases to the carpus usually have bony disease elsewhere and a life expectancy under 6 months. The lesions are often osteolytic on plain radiographs, and may be confused with an infectious or inflammatory processes if the patient's clinical history is not considered. Treatment is directed at symptomatic relief, with either tumor resection or amputation. Radiotherapy may cause fibrosis and stiffness more severe than the scarring associated with surgery.

Summary

Aside from trauma, pain or deformity are the most common concerns that prompt a consultation with a hand surgeon. Vigilance and an awareness of possible "second order" metabolic or neoplastic causes of symptoms may allow the hand surgeon to make a timely and potentially important diagnosis of underlying disease.

References

[1] Schrank C, Meirer R, Stabler A, et al. Morphology and topography of intraosseous ganglion cysts in the carpus: an anatomic, histopathologic, and magnetic resonance imaging correlation study. J Hand Surg [Am] 2003;28(1):52–61.

[2] Van den Dungen S, Marchesi S, Ezzedine R, et al. Relationship between dorsal ganglion cysts of the wrist and intraosseous ganglion cysts of the carpal bones. Acta Orthop Belg 2005;71(5):535–9 [in French].

[3] Kligman M, Roffman M. Bilateral intraosseous ganglia of the scaphoid and lunate bones. J Hand Surg [Br] 1997;22(6):820–1.

[4] Albaladejo Mora F, Sarabia Condes JM, Saura Sanchez E, et al. Intraosseous ganglion of carpal scaphoid: a case report. J Hand Surg [Am] 1993;18(4):665–6.

[5] De Smet L, Van Ransbeeck H. Intraosseous ganglion of the triquetrum. A transpisiformal approach. Acta Orthop Belg 2000;66(2):194–6 [in French].

[6] Helal B, Vernon-Roberts B. Intraosseous ganglion of the pisiform bone. Hand 1976;8(2):150–4.

[7] Ikeda M, Oka Y. Cystic lesion in carpal bone. Hand Surg 2000;5(1):25–32.

[8] Iwahara T, Hirayama T, Takemitu Y. Intraosseous ganglion of the lunate. Hand 1983;15(3):297–9.

[9] Logan SE, Gilula LA, Kyriakos M. Bilateral scaphoid ganglion cysts in an adolescent. J Hand Surg [Am] 1992;17(3):490–5.

[10] Mogan JV, Newberg AH, Davis PH. Intraosseous ganglion of the lunate. J Hand Surg [Am] 1981;6(1):61–3.

[11] Schajowicz F, Clavel Sainz M, Slullitel JA. Juxta-articular bone cysts (intra-osseous ganglia): a clinico-pathological study of eighty-eight cases. J Bone Joint Surg Br 1979;61(1):107–16.

[12] Daly PJ, Sim FH, Beabout JW, et al. Intraosseous ganglion cysts. Orthopedics 1988;11(12):1715–9.

[13] Landells JW. The bone cysts of osteoarthritis. J Bone Joint Surg Br 1953;35-B(4):643–9.

[14] Byers PD. Solitary benign osteoblastic lesions of bone. Osteoid osteoma and benign osteoblastoma. Cancer 1968;22(1):43–57.

[15] Arazi M, Memik R, Yel M, et al. Osteoid osteoma of the carpal bones. Arch Orthop Trauma Surg 2001;121(1–2):119–20.

[16] Ghiam GF, Bora FW Jr. Osteoid osteoma of the carpal bones. J Hand Surg [Am] 1978;3(3):280–3.

[17] Herndon JH, Eaton RG, Littler JW. Carpal-tunnel syndrome. An unusual presentation of osteoid-osteoma of the capitate. J Bone Joint Surg Am 1974;56(8):1715–8.

[18] De Smet L. Subperiosteal osteoid osteoma of the triquetrum mimicking an avascular necrosis. Chir Main 2002;21(2):140–2.

[19] Kernohan J, Beacon JP, Dakin PK, et al. Osteoid osteoma of the pisiform. J Hand Surg [Br] 1985;10(3):411–4.

[20] De Smet L, Fabry G. Osteoid osteoma of the hand and carpus: peculiar presentations and imaging. Acta Orthop Belg 1995;61(2):113–6 [in French].

[21] Alcalay M, Clarac JP, Bontoux D. Double osteoid-osteoma in adjacent carpal bones. A case report. J Bone Joint Surg Am 1982;64(5):779–80.

[22] Lisanti M, Rosati M, Spagnolli G, et al. Osteoid osteoma of the carpus. Case reports and a review of the literature. Acta Orthop Belg 1996;62(4):195–9 [in French].

[23] Niamane R, Lespessailles E, Deluzarches P, et al. Osteoid osteoma multifocally located and recurrent in the carpus. Joint Bone Spine 2002;69(3):327–30.

[24] Soong M, Jupiter J, Rosenthal D. Radiofrequency ablation of osteoid osteoma in the upper extremity. J Hand Surg [Am] 2006;31(2):279–83.

[25] Noble J, Lamb DW. Enchondromata of bones of the hand. A review of 40 cases. Hand 1974;6(3):275–84.

[26] Takigawa K. Chondroma of the bones of the hand. A review of 110 cases. J Bone Joint Surg Am 1971;53(8):1591–600.

[27] Emecheta IE, Bernhards J, Berger A. Carpal enchondroma. J Hand Surg [Br] 1997;22(6):817–9.

[28] Malizos KN, Gelalis ID, Ioachim EE, et al. Pathologic fracture of the scaphoid due to enchondroma: treatment with vascularized bone grafting. report of a case. J Hand Surg [Am] 1998;23(2):334–7.

[29] Minkowitz B, Patel M, Minkowitz S. Scaphoid enchondroma. Orthop Rev 1992;21(10):1241–2 1244–5.

[30] Redfern DR, Forester AJ, Evans MJ, et al. Enchondroma of the scaphoid. J Hand Surg [Br] 1997;22(2):235–6.

[31] Takka S, Poyraz A. Enchondroma of the scaphoid bone. Arch Orthop Trauma Surg 2002;122(6):369–70.

[32] Gahhos F, Cuono CB. Periosteal chondroma: another cause of carpal tunnel syndrome. Ann Plast Surg 1984;12(3):275–8.

[33] Averill RM, Smith RJ, Campbell CJ. Giant-cell tumors of the bones of the hand. J Hand Surg [Am] 1980;5(1):39–50.

[34] Weiner SD, Leeson MC. Giant cell tumor of the carpal trapezium. Orthopedics 1995;18(5):482–4.

[35] Lane CS, Kuschner SH, Mirra JM. Giant cell tumors in carpal bones. Orthopedics 1994;17(2):181–5.

[36] Howard FM, Lassen K. Giant cell tumor of the capitate. J Hand Surg [Am] 1984;9(2):272–4.

[37] Louis DS, Hankin FM, Braunstein EM. Giant cell tumour of the triquetrum. J Hand Surg [Br] 1986;11(2):279–80.

[38] FitzPatrick DJ, Bullough PG. Giant cell tumor of the lunate bone: a case report. J Hand Surg [Am] 1977;2(4):269–70.

[39] Minami A, Kato H, Iwasaki N. Vascularized fibular graft after excision of giant-cell tumor of the distal radius: wrist arthroplasty versus partial wrist arthrodesis. Plast Reconstr Surg 2002;110(1):112–7.

[40] Muramatsu K, Ihara K, Azuma E, et al. Free vascularized fibula grafting for reconstruction of the wrist following wide tumor excision. Microsurgery 2005; 25(2):101–6.

[41] Ono H, Yajima H, Mizumoto S, et al. Vascularized fibular graft for reconstruction of the wrist after excision of giant cell tumor. Plast Reconstr Surg 1997; 99(4):1086–93.

[42] Bajec J, Gang RK. Bone reconstruction with a free vascularized fibular graft after giant cell tumour resection. J Hand Surg [Br] 1993;18(5):565–7.

[43] Pho RW. Malignant giant-cell tumor of the distal end of the radius treated by a free vascularized fibular transplant. J Bone Joint Surg Am 1981;63(6):877–84.

[44] Schajowicz F, Gallardo H. Epiphysial chondroblastoma of bone. A clinico-pathological study of sixty-nine cases. J Bone Joint Surg Br 1970;52(2):205–26.

[45] Blair WF, Robinson RA, Buckwalter JA. Chondromyxoid fibroma in a carpal bone. Clin Orthop Relat Res 1984;188:199–202.

[46] Menon J, Rankin D, Jacobson C. Recurrent osteoblastoma of the carpal hamate. Orthopedics 1988; 11(4):609–11.

[47] Xarchas KC, Leviet D. Osteoblastoma of the carpal scaphoid frequency and treatment. Acta Orthop Belg 2002;68(5):532–6 [in French].

[48] Medlar RC, Sprague HH. Osteochondroma of the carpal scaphoid. J Hand Surg [Am] 1979;4(2):150–1.

[49] Rice J, Stephens M, Colville J. Scaphoid osteochondroma mimicking carpal coalition. J Hand Surg [Br] 1996;21(6):779–80.

[50] Tillman BP, Dahlin DC, Lipscomb PR, et al. Aneurysmal bone cyst: an analysis of ninety-five cases. Mayo Clin Proc 1968;43(7):478–95.

[51] Frassica FJ, Amadio PC, Wold LE, et al. Aneurysmal bone cyst: clinicopathologic features and treatment of ten cases involving the hand. J Hand Surg [Am] 1988;13(5):676–83.

[52] Moore JR, Weiland AJ, Curtis RM. Localized nodular tenosynovitis: experience with 115 cases. J Hand Surg [Am] 1984;9(3):412–7.

[53] Nilsonne U, Moberger G. Pigmented villonodular synovitis of joints. Histological and clinical problems in diagnosis. Acta Orthop Scand 1969;40(4): 448–60.

[54] Byers PD, Cotton RE, Deacon OW, et al. The diagnosis and treatment of pigmented villonodular synovitis. J Bone Joint Surg Br 1968;50(2):290–305.

[55] Carpintero P, Serrano J, Garcia-Frasquet A. Pigmented villonodular synovitis of the wrist invading bone—a report of 2 cases. Acta Orthop Scand 2000;71(4):424–6.

[56] Patel MR, Zinberg EM. Pigmented villonodular synovitis of the wrist invading bone–report of a case. J Hand Surg [Am] 1984;9(6):854–8.

[57] Schajowicz F, Blumenfeld I. Pigmented villonodular synovitis of the wrist with penetration into bone. J Bone Joint Surg Br 1968;50(2):312–3.

[58] Schwartz GB, Coleman DA. Pigmented villonodular synovitis of the wrist and adjacent bones. Orthop Rev 1986;15(8):526–30.

[59] Moynagh PD, Lettin AW. Pigmented villonodular synovitis of the wrist joint. Proc R Soc Med 1968; 61(7):670–2.

[60] Chidgey LK, Szabo RM, Wiese DA. Acute carpal tunnel syndrome caused by pigmented villonodular synovitis of the wrist. Clin Orthop Relat Res 1988; 228:254–7.

[61] Loonen MP, Schuurman AH. Recurrent synovial chondromatosis of the wrist: case report and literature review. Acta Orthop Belg 2005;71(2):230–5 [in French].

[62] Rompen JC, Ham SJ, Molenaar WM, et al. Synovial chondromatosis of the wrist and hand—a case report. Acta Orthop Scand 1999;70(6):627–9.

[63] Ono H, Yajima H, Fukui A, et al. Locking wrist with synovial chondromatosis: report of two cases. J Hand Surg [Am] 1994;19(5):797–9.

[64] Marcuzzi A, Maiorana A, Adani R, et al. Osteosarcoma of the scaphoid. A case report and review of the literature. J Bone Joint Surg Br 1996;78(5):699–701.

[65] Bickerstaff DR, Harris SC, Kay NR. Osteosarcoma of the carpus. J Hand Surg [Br] 1988;13(3):303–5.

[66] Dahlin DC, Salvador AH. Chondrosarcomas of bones of the hands and feet—a study of 30 cases. Cancer 1974;34(3):755–60.

[67] Granberry WM, Bryan W. Chondrosarcoma of the trapezium: a case report. J Hand Surg [Am] 1978; 3(3):277–9.

[68] Kerin R. The hand in metastatic disease. J Hand Surg [Am] 1987;12(1):77–83.

[69] Wu KK, Guise ER. Metastatic tumors of the hand: a report of six cases. J Hand Surg [Am] 1978;3(3): 271–6.

[70] Craigen MA, Chesney RB. Metastatic adenocarcinoma of the carpus: a case report. J Hand Surg [Br] 1988;13(3):306–7.

[71] Cary PC, Helms CA, Genant HK. Metastatic disease to the carpus. Br J Radiol 1981;54(647):992–5.

[72] Cohen HJ, Laszlo J. Influence of trauma on the unusual distribution of metastases from carcinoma of the larynx. Cancer 1972;29(2):466–71.

[73] Gold GL, Reefe WE. Carcinoma and metastases to the bones of the hand. JAMA 1963;184:237–9.

[74] Dolich BH, Spinner M, Kaufman G. Isolated metastasis to the carpal bones. Report of a case. Bull Hosp Joint Dis 1970;31(1):78–84.

[75] Gottlieb PD, Parikh SJ, Singh JK. Case report 295. Metastatic disease of the carpus (primary site: bronchogenic carcinoma). Skeletal Radiol 1985;13(2): 154–8.

[76] Smith RJ. Involvement of the carpal bones with metastatic tumor. Am J Roentgenol Radium Ther Nucl Med 1963;89:1253–5.

[77] Ioia JV, Sumner JM, Gallagher T. Presentation of malignancy by metastasis to the carpal navicular bone. Clin Orthop Relat Res 1984;(188):230–3.

[78] Kerin R. Metastatic tumors of the hand. J Bone Joint Surg Am 1958;40-A(2):263–77 [discussion: 277–8].

[79] Kerin R. Metastatic tumors of the hand. A review of the literature. J Bone Joint Surg Am 1983;65(9): 1331–5.

ELSEVIER
SAUNDERS

Hand Clin 22 (2006) 447–463

HAND
CLINICS

Disorders of the Immature Carpus

Patricia A. Hsu, MD, Terry R. Light, MD*

Loyola Department of Orthopaedic Surgery and Rehabilitation, 2160 South First Avenue, Maguire, Room 1700, Maywood, IL 60153, USA

Carpal disorders in children are often associated with developmental abnormalities of structures surrounding the wrist. Conditions that alter the function and position of the arm, forearm, and hand will also ultimately influence carpal development and function. Because the immature carpus is composed of unossified cartilage, carpal abnormalities in young children are frequently undetectable on plain radiographs. Over time, the carpus ossifies and the abnormalities become evident. Clinical suspicion of an abnormality may elicit further imaging with MRI, which can provide detailed information about cartilaginous structures.

Development

The carpal bones develop from mesenchymal cells located within the deep layer of the limb bud mesoderm. The mesenchymal cells initially form an extracellular matrix that establishes the cartilaginous primordium of the skeleton. By the sixth week of gestation, this matrix has differentiated into the cartilage model of the humerus, ulna, radius, metacarpals, and proximal phalanges. By the eighth week, histologic sections show early carpal and joint definition (Fig. 1), with complete joint definition by 10.5 weeks (Fig. 2) [1].

At birth, the carpal bones are entirely cartilaginous. Each bone ossifies postnatally through sequential centripetal expansion. The ossific nucleus of the capitate may be visible as early as 6 weeks after birth, and is usually present by the

third to fourth month when the ossific nucleus of the hamate also begins to appear. The nucleus of the triquetrum appears between the seventh and 24th month. The lunate becomes visible between ages 3 and 4 years. The trapezium, trapezoid, and scaphoid develop their ossific nuclei between ages 3 and 6 years, typically appearing in that order. The pisiform is the last carpal bone to become visible on radiograph, with its ossific nucleus appearing between ages 8 and 12 years. The carpal bones typically attain full maturity between the 14th and 18th postnatal year [2]. Immature incompletely ossified cartilaginous carpi can be visualized with MRI.

Bipartite carpal bones

Carpal bones usually ossify through centripetal expansion from a single ossific nucleus. Occasionally, ossification will occur from two separate nuclei that coalesce with maturation. Failure of two separate ossific nuclei to coalesce may lead to a bipartite carpal bone [3].

The scaphoid is the most frequently reported congenitally bipartite carpal bone. Gruber and Pfitzner [4–6] first described a bipartite scaphoid through anatomic studies in the late 1900s. However, the validity of these early reports has been questioned because the authors used lye during specimen preparation, which removed all cartilaginous tissue. Without observing cartilage between the bipartite segments, researchers argue that a congenitally bipartite scaphoid could not truly be distinguished from an occult scaphoid nonunion [7].

Although select case reports of bipartite scaphoids exist [8], their incidence is extremely rare, estimated by Louis and colleagues [7] to be approximately 0.00017%. In an effort to aid in

---

* Corresponding author.
E-mail address: tlight@lumc.edu (T.R. Light).

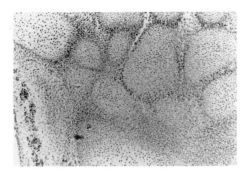

Fig. 1. Histologic section of carpus at 8 weeks showing early carpal and joint definition. (*From* Light TR. Growth and development of the hand. In: Carter PR, editor. Reconstruction of the child's hand. Philadelphia: Lea & Febiger; 1990. p. 116; with permission.)

the diagnosis of congenital bipartite scaphoid, Bunnell [7,9] outlined several supportive criteria, including

1. Absence of a history of trauma
2. Presence of bilateral scaphoid bipartition
3. Equal size/density of both ossicles
4. Absence of degenerative changes in the radial scaphoid carpal articulation
5. Presence of a clear space between the components with smooth edges at the joint surfaces

Although any or all of these criteria do not definitively confirm the presence of a true congenital bipartite scaphoid, they can be used with a patient's history and symptoms to at least consider congenital bipartite scaphoid as a possible, albeit rare, diagnosis.

Carpal coalition

Carpal coalitions are the result of incomplete or absent joint formation between cartilaginous carpal precursors. Case reports have documented coalition between virtually every combination of adjacent carpal bones (Fig. 3A,B). In addition, radiocarpal and carpometacarpal fusions have been documented. Lunatotriquetral fusion is the most common carpal coalition, with an incidence of approximately 0.1% (Fig. 4) [10], followed by capitohamate fusions. Because the carpus ossifies throughout childhood, coalitions are rarely radiologically evident until adolescence.

Coalition can manifest as part of a congenital syndrome, such as one listed in Box 1, or as an isolated abnormality. Coalitions associated with syndromes often involve more than two bones

and may bridge the proximal and distal rows. Although wrist motion may be limited, no treatment is indicated. Isolated coalitions usually occur within the same row and affect only two bones [11]. Most isolated carpal coalitions are asymptomatic and present as incidental findings on radiographs.

Incomplete development of intercarpal joints may result in an incomplete coalition with an osseous bridge between bones. With stress, these unstable joints may develop painful synovitis. Symptomatic carpal coalition has also been reported in patients who have incomplete fusions resembling pseudarthrosis [11]. The lunatotriquetral joint, which is the joint most commonly involved in a total synostosis, is also the joint that is most often symptomatic secondary to incomplete fusion. Diagnosis of coalition may not be possible with plain films alone; a CT scan may be necessary to visualize any subtle bony bridging. Bone scan may also be useful to show increased radionuclide uptake at the affected joint.

A symptomatic incomplete carpal coalition is effectively treated by fusing the involved joint. Any remaining cartilage should be curettaged from the joint to expose subchondral bone. Autogenous bone graft from the ipsilateral distal radius is packed into the interval to supplement the fusion. Internal fixation and immobilization may be used to increase the likelihood of complete joint fusion. Lunatotriquetral fusion results in minimal loss of wrist motion [3].

Recent case reports have described ulnar neuropathy associated with pisiform–hamate coalition. Both patients treated by Berkowitz and

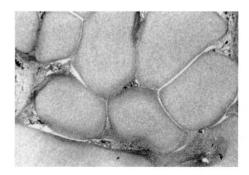

Fig. 2. Histologic section of carpus at 10.5 weeks showing intercarpal joint definition with continuity of soft tissue attachments. (*From* Light TR. Growth and development of the hand. In: Carter PR, editor. Reconstruction of the child's hand. Philadelphia: Lea & Febiger; 1990. p. 117; with permission.)

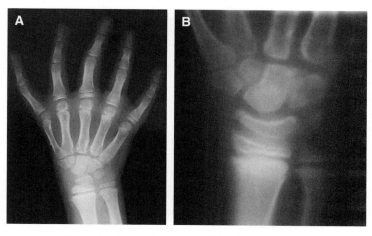

Fig. 3. (*A, B*) Scapholunate coalition in pentadactyly.

Melone [15] showed a large bony prominence over the pisiform and an enlarged hook of the hamate in addition to the coalition. Symptoms resolved after operative decompression of the ulnar nerve in Guyon's canal. Fracture through lunotriquetral coalitions have also been reported, but are rare [16].

Accessory carpal bones

Because true accessory carpal bones are uncommon, with an incidence of 0.4%–1.6% [17,18], these small bones are often mistaken for fractures of normal carpal bones [2,19,20]. Accessoria have been given various names (eg, os triangulare, os epitriquetrum, os hypotriquetrum, os lunatotriquetrum, os centrale, os ulnostyloideum) to reflect either the shape or presumed phylogenic derivation of the bone [2]. Disorders that have been associated with accessory carpals include Holt-Oram syndrome [21], hand-foot-uterus syndrome, Larsen's syndrome, and otopalatodigital complex [2]. Accessory carpal bones have also been found in otherwise healthy nonsyndromic patients [19,22].

Accessory carpal bones are generally asymptomatic. However, they may occasionally cause painful swelling, clicking, and crepitus [2,19,23]. Koizumi and colleagues [24] recently documented a case of attritional rupture of the index finger flexor digitorum profundus tendon caused by an accessory carpal bone located palmar to the capitate and triquetrum. Symptomatic patients can be treated with short-term splinting [22]. If

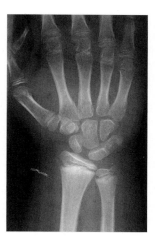

Fig. 4. Congenital lunatotriquetral fusion.

> **Box 1. Syndromes associated with carpal coalition [2,12–14]**
>
> Arthrogryposis multiplex congenita
> Hereditary symphalangism associated
>   with carpal and tarsal fusion
> Hand-foot-uterus syndrome
> Apert syndrome
> Acro-pectoro-vertebral dysplasia
> Ellis-van Creveld syndrome
>   (chondroectodermal dysplasia)
> Holt-Oram syndrome
> Otopalatodigital syndrome
> Diastrophic dwarfism
> Turner's syndrome
> Dyschondrosteosis
> Bird-headed dwarfism

symptoms persist, the accessory bone may be removed through either arthroscopic or open resection [19,23].

Absences

Congenital absences of carpal bones are usually associated with disorders such as radial and ulnar ray deficiency, cleft hand, phocomelia, and ulnar dimelia [2]. Although a few cases have been documented [25–29], true isolated absences of carpal bones are rare. Several past reports of presumed isolated absences have since been classified into a group of malformations known as *intercalary radial hemimelia* [17]. Characteristics include absence of the scaphoid, occasional absence of the trapezium, and developmental defects of the radial styloid, thumb ray, and thenar muscles [25]. Treble [30] documented a case of congenital absence of the scaphoid in a patient who had VATER syndrome. This patient also had absence of the radial styloid and hypoplasia of the trapezium and thumb metacarpal, making a diagnosis of intercalary radial hemimelia more likely.

Recently, carpal absence associated with ectrodactyly was attributed to mild forms of radial and ulnar longitudinal deficiency. In 1999, James and colleagues [31] modified the Bayne and Klug [32] classification of radial deficiency to include a type 0 precursor, defined as a hypoplastic or absent thumb and absent, hypoplastic, or coalesced carpal bones in the presence of a normal radius. Havenhill and colleagues [33] also made a similar modification to the Bayne [34] classification of ulnar longitudinal deficiency (ULD) to include ulnar-sided hand deficiencies without forearm or elbow involvement. The ULD type 0 precursor is defined as hypoplastic or absent ring and small fingers, absent/hypoplastic/coalesced carpal bones, and a normal-length ulna [33].

Arthrogryposis multiplex congenita

Arthrogryposis is characterized by multiple congenital joint contractures and hypoplastic musculature. Although the cause is unknown, several theories have been proposed, including viral infection of the central nervous system, anterior horn cell degeneration, and embryonic arrest of muscle development [35]. Conditions such as oligohydramnios and increased intrauterine pressure, which result in decreased embryonic movement in utero, have also been suggested as possible contributing factors. Administering

paralytic agents in chick embryos has been shown to cause multiple joint contractures, providing support for intrauterine theories [36].

Clinical presentations of arthrogryposis can be broadly categorized into two forms. Neuropathic arthrogryposis accounts for 90% of cases and is characterized by either fixed flexion or extension contractures of the limbs [3], whereas the less-common myopathic form is characterized by hypotonia and hyporeflexia with or without the presence of contractures and is more often accompanied by chest and spine abnormalities [3,37]. Typical upper-extremity contractures in arthrogryposis include adduction and internal rotation of the shoulder, flexion or extension of the elbow, forearm pronation, and wrist flexion with ulnar deviation. A thumb-in-palm deformity is often seen with associated narrowing of the first web space.

The carpal bones frequently coalesce into a single osseous mass that, in combination with wrist flexion contracture, limits wrist motion. The extent of wrist contractures caused by arthrogryposis does not increase postnatally. Most cases are bilateral, with distal limb structures showing the greatest deformity [37].

Affected children are remarkably resourceful in adapting to their deformity. Many use a bimanual crossover grip to pick up objects. Although simple machines have been devised to aid with feeding in the arthrogrypotic position, personal hygiene remains problematic because only the dorsum of the hand can reach the perineum [38]. Treatment of the upper extremities in children who have arthrogryposis focuses on achieving the ability to perform these essential activities of daily living.

In younger children, soft tissue release alone may provide adequate correction of wrist flexion. The flexor carpi ulnaris, flexor carpi radialis, palmaris longus, and palmar fascia may all be released to decrease wrist flexion [39]. This technique can be supplemented with a tendon transfer of the flexor carpi ulnaris to the dorsum of the wrist for improved soft tissue balance [39,40].

When soft tissue modifications alone do not provide sufficient improvement, surgical alteration of the carpus or the distal radius may become necessary to increase passive wrist dorsiflexion. If the proximal and distal carpal rows have not coalesced, proximal row carpectomy may be performed to improve dorsiflexion [41]. If only a single coalesced carpal mass is present, a dorsal carpal closing wedge osteotomy may be performed instead [3].

In patients nearing skeletal maturity, wrist flexion contracture may be treated with either a dorsal closing wedge osteotomy of the distal radius [42] or a wrist fusion [3]. If the carpus has not entirely coalesced, proximal row carpectomy and fusion of the capitate to the radius with bone graft from the excised carpal bones may be performed to achieve wrist arthrodesis. In the more common case of a single osseous carpal mass, a dorsal wedge removed from the radiocarpal junction will facilitate fusion between the decorticated carpal mass and distal radius [38].

Carpal tarsal osteolysis

Carpal tarsal osteolysis (CTO) is an uncommon condition characterized by the spontaneous resorption of the carpal bones (Fig. 5). Although the cause of osteolysis is still unknown, the condition has shown both autosomal dominant and recessive inheritance patterns in addition to spontaneous occurrence [43]. Several physical findings may be associated with CTO, including abnormal skull shape, micrognathia, high-arched palate, decreased height, and scoliosis [44]. CTO is also frequently associated with renal dysfunction, which is the leading cause of mortality in affected patients [45,46].

Children who have carpal tarsal osteolysis have normal cartilaginous carpal precursors in infancy. As the carpus begins to ossify between ages 2 and 5 years, CTO presents as an acute arthritis with swelling of the wrists and ankles followed by a period of slow, painless osteolysis [47]. Often misdiagnosed as juvenile rheumatoid arthritis (JRA), CTO can be distinguished from JRA based on a the absence of (1) elevated acute phase reactants, (2) inflammatory change on biopsy specimens, and (3) characteristic radiographic findings for JRA (ie, thickened cortices of carpals and phalanges caused by periosteal changes, true subchondral erosion, and spontaneous bony fusion) [48].

No definitive treatment currently exists for CTO. Nonsteroidal anti-inflammatory drugs (NSAIDs) can be administered for analgesia during painful episodes, and physical therapy and splints worn for stabilization can provide some relief during symptomatic periods and help maintain functional positions, but they do not influence the progression of the disease [47]. Over time, the entire carpus may be resorbed, resulting in gross instability and dislocation of the hand (Fig. 6). Although the wrist is unstable, extrinsic and intrinsic musculotendinous function is preserved, as is active flexion and extension of the metacarpophalangeal and interphalangeal joints. Manual dexterity may remain surprisingly functional, albeit weak, and surgery is rarely indicated [3].

Dysplasia epiphysealis hemimelica (Trevor disease)

Dysplasia epiphysealis hemimelica (DEH), or Trevor disease, is a developmental disorder of unknown origin characterized by osteocartilaginous

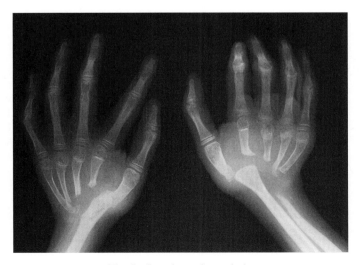

Fig. 5. Carpal tarsal osteolysis.

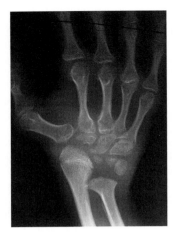

Fig. 6. Radiocarpal dislocation in a patient who has Morquio's wrist.

overgrowth of one or more epiphyses. Common sites of presentation include the distal tibia, distal femur, and talus [49–52]. Although upper extremity involvement is rare, several cases of DEH were reported involving the radius, ulna, and carpus (Fig. 7A,B) [53–58]. Symptoms from DEH include restricted range of motion and pain caused by deformity of the joint involved. Taniguchi and Tamaki [54] reported a case of DEH affecting the ipsilateral scaphoid and trapezium of a 9-year-old girl, resulting in scapholunate dissociation and carpal instability. In mild cases, carpal DEH may be treated with splinting [53]. For more severe cases, resection of the impinging carpal or radial bone may be necessary to restore motion [3].

Ulnar dimelia

Ulnar dimelia is a very rare congenital abnormality with approximately 60 cases documented worldwide [59]. Also known as "mirror hand," the forearm and hand are essentially symmetrical about the mid-line with duplication of the ulna and ulna rays and an absence of the radius and radial rays. The condition is typically unilateral, although instances of bilateral ulnar dimelia have been documented [60,61].

No specific genetic abnormality has been linked to ulnar dimelia. Spontaneous mutation has been suggested as a possible cause [59]. Regarding embryogenesis, Gorriz [62] explained the development of ulnar dimelia as a failure of complete anteroposterior differentiation of the limb bud rather than a true ulnar duplication. Chinegwundoh and colleagues [59] support this theory, directing their attention toward the ability of the preaxial ulna to mature into a near-normal distal radius.

The preaxial ulna is often broader than a normal ulna, resembling a normal distal radius. Ulnar dimelia is characterized by the absence of the thumb, scaphoid, and trapezium. The hand consists of seven or eight digits, with the radial digits performing the function of opposition as a group. Duplication of the remaining carpal bones (ie, pisiform, triquetrum, hamate, capitate, and lunate) also occurs in a symmetrical fashion [63]. The proximal row contains two triquetral bones, each articulating with its own pisiform. An abnormally wide lunate formed from two lunate bones fused side-by-side sits in the center of the proximal

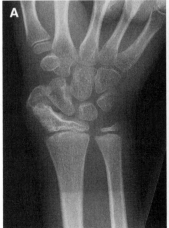
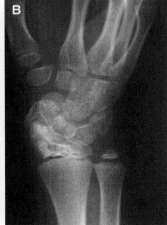

Fig. 7. (*A, B*) Dysplasia epiphysealis hemimelica/Trevor disease affecting the distal radius and scaphoid.

row. The distal row usually consists of two ha-mate and two capitate bones articulating with each other at the midline. A single bone which may represent a trapezoid is sometimes present between the two capitate [63].

Several abnormalities are also present in the forearm. At the elbow, the distal humerus lacks a capitellum and is composed of two ill-defined trochleas. Elbow flexion and extension are limited by the degree of joint abnormality. Forearm rotation is impossible because of the absence of proximal and distal radioulnar joints [64]. In addition, the wrist is often fixed in a flexed posture partly because of the relative abundance of flexor muscles and lack of extensors [3].

Surgical treatment of ulnar dimelia should address limitations of elbow flexion, wrist contracture, and digital excess. Pollicization of one of the preaxial digits, deletion of the remaining supernumerary preaxial digits, and reinforcement with muscle and tendon taken from the deleted digits help normalize the appearance of the hand [65].

The flexion contracture at the wrist reflects excessive flexor forces and can be addressed with several procedures, including proximal muscle release, distal tenotomy, volar wrist capsulotomy, and proximal row carpectomy [65]. Tendon transfer from the volar to the dorsal aspect of the hand may be necessary to maintain a corrected wrist posture through increasing active wrist extension [62]. Although resection of the proximal ulna has been suggested as a means of improving elbow motion and forearm rotation, long-term preservation of the motion achieved has been variable [66].

Because these forearms lack an interosseous membrane, resection of the proximal preaxial ulna may allow the remaining ulna to migrate proximally, which may then lead to further abnormalities in carpal posture and wrist motion.

Multiple hereditary exostoses

Multiple hereditary exostoses (MHE) is a benign autosomal dominant skeletal dysplasia that typically presents in the first decade of life [67]. In children, early exostoses appear as asymmetrical overgrowths of the cortex adjacent to a physis (Fig. 8A, B). Because these lesions are partially cartilaginous, MRI may be needed to accurately determine their size and location [68].

The forearm is affected in approximately 60% of patients who have MHE [68]. When the ulna is affected, its longitudinal growth decreases [3]. Presence of an involved shortened ulna typically results in ulnar bowing of the distal radius, ulnar translation of the carpus, and dislocation of the radial head [67]. Because the relative shortening of the ulna contributes to most wrist and elbow deformity in MHE, surgical intervention is directed at either lengthening the ulna or releasing its tether to the carpus and distal radius.

Ulnar lengthening may be performed with either a single-stage sliding step-cut osteotomy [69] or through gradual lengthening with either an Ilizarov or a uniplanar device [70–72]. If the ulna is lengthened when the patient is far from skeletal maturity, relative shortening of the ulna may recur [3]. Alternatively, the ulnar collateral ligament

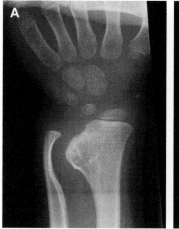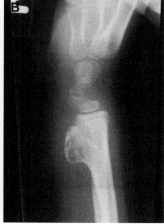

Fig. 8. (*A, B*) Multiple hereditary exostosis of the distal radius.

may be released at its carpal insertion, effectively disengaging the carpus from the ulna [73].

Lesions of the distal radius and ulna resulting in symptomatic impingement may also be resected. Cases of excessive radial inclination may be corrected through stapling the radial aspect of the distal radial physis [74].

Madelung's deformity

Madelung's deformity reflects asymmetric growth of the distal radial physis. As the radial and dorsal portions of the physis continue to grow, several abnormalities manifest. Increased palmar and ulnar tilt of the distal radial articular surface leads to volar translation of the hand and wrist. Although the reduction of growth is most prominent along the ulnar and volar distal radial physis, an overall reduction of growth occurs along the entire physis compared with normal, resulting in a shortened radius. The distal ulnar physis remains affected and continues to grow, causing incongruity of the distal radioulnar joint and dorsal subluxation of the ulnar head.

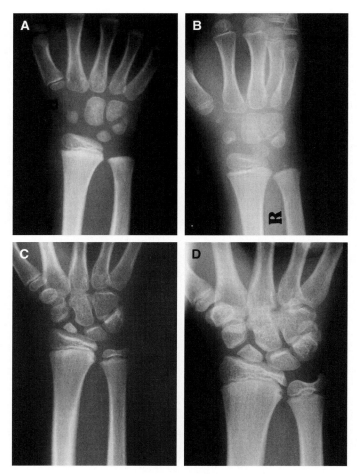

Fig. 9. Closed crush injury in a 5.75-year-old boy resulting in fractures of the triquetrum and scaphoid. (*A*) Radiograph at injury showing a fracture of the triquetrum. No radiographic evidence of injury to the scaphoid is present. (*B*) Healing of the triquetrum is evident 3 months after injury. An area of sclerosis and cupping is present at the proximal edge of the scaphoid ossification center. (*C*) Nonunion of the scaphoid is radiographically evident 3 years after injury. There is a difference in density between the proximal and distal ossification centers of the scaphoid. (*D*) Nonunion of the scaphoid persists 4 years after injury. Bone density is now similar in the proximal and distal ossification centers. (*From* Larson B, Light TR, Ogden JA. Fracture and ischemic necrosis of the immature scaphoid. J Hand Surg [Am] 1987;12(1): 123–4. Copyright © 1987, with permission from The American Society for Surgery of the Hand.)

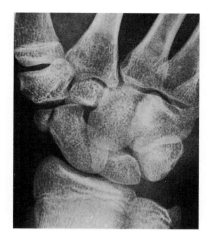

Fig. 10. Avulsion injury of the distal pole of the scaphoid in an adolescent patient. (*From:* Beatty E, Light TR, Belsole RJ, et al. Wrist and hand skeletal injuries in children. Hand Clin 1990;6(4):725; with permission.)

The carpal contour is distorted. The normal curved shape of the proximal carpal row molds itself into a peaked V-shape over time to match the defect in the distal radioulnar articular surface. As the carpus migrates proximally into the defect, the distal radius and ulna are splayed apart. The anatomic changes result in decreased range of motion, decreased grip strength, wrist pain, and poor cosmesis [3,75].

Henry and Thorburn [76] classified Madelung's deformity into four different etiologic groups: (1) idiopathic or primary, (2) secondary to trauma, infection, or tumor, (3) dysplastic, including skeletal dysplasias, and (4) genetic, including Turner's syndrome [75]. Idiopathic Madelung's deformity shows autosomal dominance with a 50% penetrance [76] and is bilateral in approximately 50% to 60% of cases [3]. The condition typically presents in adolescent women who complain of increasing wrist deformity. Occasionally an atypical Madelung's deformity develops from premature arrest of the radial and dorsal portions of the distal radial physis, resulting in a reversed pattern of deformity [3].

Several surgical interventions exist for treating Madelung's deformity. Vickers and colleagues [77] were the first to notice an abnormal fibrous ligament tethering the distal radius to the carpal bones along the volar surface, primarily the lunate, and proposed that resecting this ligament may assist carpal advancement. Carter and Ezaki [78] reviewed the results of 23 wrists treated with distal radial dome osteotomy and release of this tethered ligament. Releasing the ligament alone was found to be effective in relieving painful symptoms even before the osteotomy had healed. These results suggest that releasing this ligament may be important not only for restoring more normal carpal–radial alignment but also for pain relief.

Younger patients who have mild to moderate deformity and substantial growth potential may benefit from epiphysiolysis, which involves excising the prematurely fused ulnar-half of the distal radial physis [3]. In older patients who have more severe deformity, various osteotomy procedures have been described to address abnormal radial inclination and relative ulnar overgrowth. Salon and colleagues [79] published late follow-up (average 9.7 years) of 11 wrists treated during adolescence with a closing wedge osteotomy of the radius, shortening osteotomy of the ulna, and conservation of the distal radioulnar joint. All wrists were pain-free with activities of daily living at final follow-up. Houshian and colleagues [75] found similar results in a group of seven patients treated with radial osteotomy and lengthening using the Ilizarov technique.

Carpal tunnel syndrome

Carpal tunnel syndrome (CTS) occurs infrequently in children. Several groups of children show increased susceptibility to CTS, including those who have lysosomal storage diseases, mucopolysaccharidoses, mucolipidoses, hemophilia, hemangiomas, macrodactyly, and familial CTS. In addition, children engaging in sports such as weight lifting and skiing are more prone to developing CTS. Most children present with complaints of clumsy hands, wrist pain, and hand pain. Older children experience symptoms similar to those of adults, including paresthesias and nocturnal pain. Physical examination of those who have systemic disease often shows marked thenar weakness and atrophy. Because pediatric cases of CTS tend to show bilateral electrophysiologic abnormalities, experts recommend that electromyography and nerve conduction studies be performed bilaterally in all children who have suspected CTS [80]. Childhood CTS has only shown effective treatment with open operative release [80].

Fracture

The scaphoid is the most commonly injured carpal bone in children, followed by the capitate

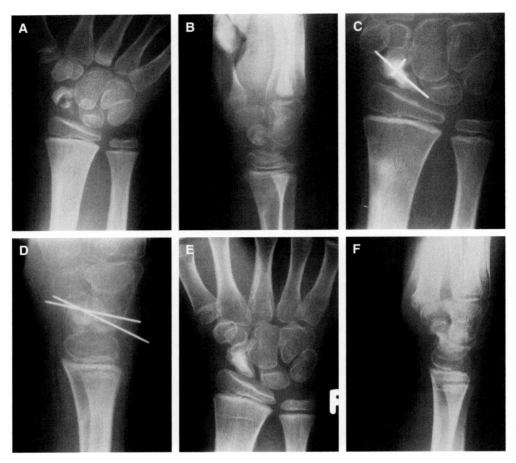

Fig. 11. (*A–F*) Pediatric scaphoid fractured treated with percutaneous pinning and bone graft. (*Courtesy of* H. K. Watson, MD, Hartford, Connecticut.)

[81]. Combined injury of these carpal bones is a well-documented entity in children and is referred to as *scaphocapitate syndrome*. The most common mechanism of injury, which is the same for children and adults, is a fall onto an outstretched hand. Because the carpus is unossified through most of childhood, MRI may be needed in addition to plain radiographs to detect injuries of the immature carpus (Fig. 9A–D) [82].

Scaphoid

The distal pole of the scaphoid ossifies before the proximal pole, resulting in an increased incidence of distal-third fractures and avulsions of the distal radial aspect of the scaphoid in children compared with adults (Fig. 10) [81,83,84]. Other patterns of injury common to the pediatric population include scaphoid fractures occurring in association with distal radius fractures, and

incomplete fractures involving only one cortex [85,86]. Most pediatric scaphoid fractures are nondisplaced and heal with 4 to 6 weeks of immobilization [81]. As in adults, displaced fractures are treated with open reduction and internal fixation (Fig. 11A–F) [87,88].

Closed treatment of an unstable scaphoid fracture may result in a humpback deformity malunion. Although this malunion predictably leads to problems in adults, including lunate dorsiflexion and limited range of motion [81], Suzuki and Herbert [89] showed that one child was able to remodel scaphoid malunion and spontaneously correct dorsal intercalated segment instability.

Capitate

Because capitate fractures are difficult to diagnose in adults and children, they are often

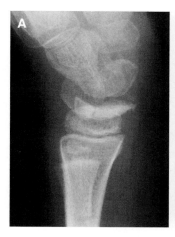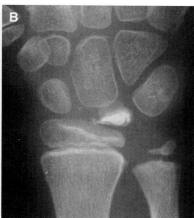

Fig. 12. (*A*, *B*) Kienböck disease in a pediatric patient. (*From* Rasmussen F, Schantz K. Lunatomalacia in a child. Acta Orthop Scand 1987;58(1):82–4; with permission.)

missed. Injury usually occurs in association with fractures of other wrist bones, most commonly the scaphoid [81]. In scaphocapitate syndrome, a fracture of the neck of the capitate is associated with a fracture of the waist of the adjacent scaphoid. Several authors have reported this combined injury in children [90–93]. Nondisplaced fractures of the capitate can be adequately treated with immobilization [94]. Displaced fractures require open or percutaneous reduction and internal fixation [92].

Kienböck's disease

Kienböck's disease usually affects adults and occurs most often in men in their 20s and 30s [81]. Although this disorder is highly uncommon in the pediatric population, children as young as 7 years of age have been diagnosed with Kienböck's disease (Fig. 12A,B) [95].

The optimal treatment of pediatric Kienböck's disease remains uncertain. Younger children have been shown to spontaneously revascularize the lunate when treated with prolonged immobilization [96]. Cases refractory to conservative measures may require surgical intervention. Unloading of the lunate through distal radial shortening with plate fixation has produced mixed results in children [97,98]. Yasuda and colleagues [99] achieved clinical improvement with percutaneous pinning of the scaphotrapezoid joint and temporary immobilization of the carpus; the pins were removed after 4 months with no permanent wrist stiffness.

Preiser's disease (scaphoid ischemic necrosis)

Although Preiser [100] has been criticized for including patients who have a history of trauma in his original 1910 publication [101], scaphoid ischemic necrosis without trauma is still commonly referred to as *Preiser's disease*. Although atraumatic ischemic necrosis of the scaphoid has been associated with systemic lupus erythematosus, systemic sclerosis, steroid ingestion, and cytotoxic chemotherapy [102–105], several cases have been reported in which no apparent cause could be identified [106–109].

Children who have thumb hypoplasia and associated radial dysplasia often have a small hypoplastic scaphoid (Fig. 13A–C). High compressive loads across the carpal joints generated by hand function and grip may lead to failure of the hypoplastic scaphoid, which is intrinsically more susceptible to ischemic necrosis and fracture [110].

Juvenile idiopathic arthritis

To consolidate terminology for classifying chronic childhood arthritis, the International League Against Rheumatism adopted the term *juvenile idiopathic arthritis (JIA)*, which encompasses the diseases previously known as *juvenile rheumatoid arthritis* and *juvenile chronic* arthritis [111]. In patients who have JIA, the wrist is a very commonly involved joint, second only to the knee, and is affected in approximately 54% to 59% of patients [112,113]. Initial radiographic

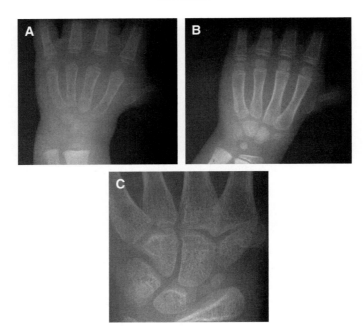

Fig. 13. (A–C) Preiser's disease (scaphoid ischemic necrosis) in a patient who has VACTERL syndrome anomalies, including scoliosis, anal atresia, tracheoesophageal fistula, and thumb hypoplasia. (Fig. 13C *from* Light TR. Injury to the immature carpus. Hand Clin 1988;4(3):421; with permission. Case provided by Neil Marcus, MD, Detroit, Michigan.)

changes include premature ossification of the carpus, narrowing of the intercarpal joint spaces, and early closure of the distal ulnar physis (Fig. 14A,B) [114]. The resulting negative ulnar variance is associated with ulnar translocation and ultimately dislocation of the carpus, described by Chaplin [112] as the "bayonet deformity."

Treatment for JIA consists mainly of drug therapy designed to attenuate the inflammatory response. Aspirin, NSAIDs, gold salts, methotrexate, hydroxychloroquine, penicillamine, and systemic corticosteroids are all currently prescribed [115]. In a study by Harel and colleagues [116], methotrexate improved wrist symptoms in 74% of patients, 65% of which showed actual improvement in carpal length on radiographs. In wrist disease that is unresponsive to medication, steroid injection is generally effective for reducing synovitis [114]. Synovectomy has also been shown to improve symptoms of boggy swollen joints, but should not be performed in patients who have minimal synovial thickening where fibrous ankylosis is already present [117]. Distraction lengthening of the shortened ulna has been proposed as a method of decreasing ulnar translation of the carpus [114]. Although the procedure has been shown to correct pre-existing deformity, its long-term effectiveness is not yet known.

Pauciarticular disease

Approximately 45% of patients who have JIA have arthritis limited to one or only a few joints. Larger joints are typically involved in a nonsymmetric distribution [115]. Pauciarticular disease is associated with ocular involvement, including anterior uveitis and chronic iridocyclitis [115,118]. Because ocular involvement does not usually present until late in the disease process, frequent eye examinations are a critical component of care. Jay and colleagues [115] recommend that children who have oligoarthritis undergo ophthalmologic examination every 3 months for the first 2 years of disease followed by biannual examinations thereafter.

Down syndrome

Very little has been written about wrist abnormalities in Down syndrome. The senior author (TRL) has treated two patients who had Down syndrome who developed nondissociative midcarpal subluxation with palmar flexion of the

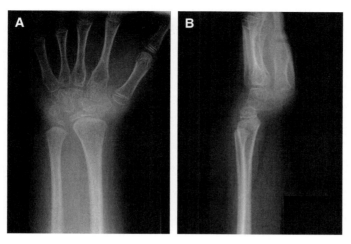

Fig. 14. (*A*, *B*) Juvenile idiopathic arthritis of the wrist.

proximal carpal row secondary to ligamentous laxity (Fig. 15A–D). One patient underwent intercarpal arthrodesis and eventually developed radiocarpal subluxation, suggesting that total wrist arthrodesis may be necessary to ensure long-term stability in patients who have this condition [81].

Summary

Congenital abnormalities of the carpus are rare in isolation and typically present as part of a generalized syndrome. Treatment of carpal disorders within these syndromes continues to require an understanding of the influence the wrist's position on overall upper extremity function. In addition, carpal ossification throughout childhood presents a unique set of influences regarding pediatric carpal injury. Although the pediatric carpus is capable of remodeling and revascularization, cases requiring surgical intervention depend on the physician's level of clinical suspicion for timely diagnosis and treatment.

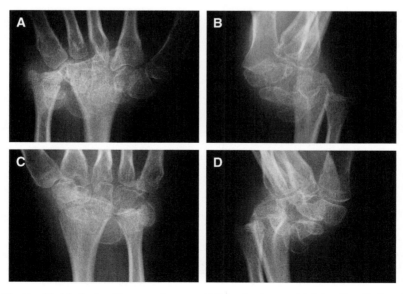

Fig. 15. (*A–D*) 14-year-old girl who has Down syndrome and bilateral palmar wrist dislocation. Patient did not have any wrist pain and was referred by her cardiologist for bilateral hand weakness.

References

[1] Light TR. Growth and development of the hand. In: Carter PR, editor. Reconstruction of the child's hand. Philadelphia: Lea & Febiger; 1990. p. 113–26.

[2] Kelikian H. Anomalies of carpal bones. Congenital deformities of the hand and forearm. Philadelphia: W. B. Saunders Company; 1974.

[3] Light TR, Janelle C. Congenital malformations. In: Herndon JH, editor. Surgical reconstruction of the upper extremity. Stamford: Appleton & Lange; 1999. p. 723–37.

[4] Gruber W. Os Naviculare carpi bipartitum. Arch Pathol Anat Physiol Klin Med 1877;69:391–6.

[5] Pfitzner W. Beitrage zur Kenntniss des menschlichen Extremitatenskelets. VI. Die Variationen in Aufbau der Handskelets. Morph Arb 1895;4: 347–570.

[6] Pfitzner W. Beitrage zur Kenntniss des menschlichen Extremitatenskelets. VIII. Die morphologischen Elemente des menschlichen Handskelets. Morph Arb 1900;2:77–157, 365–678.

[7] Louis DS, Calhoun TP, Garn SM, et al. Congenital bipartite scaphoid—fact or fiction? J Bone Joint Surg Am 1976;58(8):1108–12.

[8] Doman AN, Marcus NW. Congenital bipartite scaphoid. J Hand Surg [Am] 1990;15(6):869–73.

[9] Bunnell S. Fractures and dislocations: injuries of the wrist. In: Boyes JH, editor. Bunnell's surgery of the hand. 5th edition. Philadelphia: J. B. Lippincott Company; 1970. p. 592.

[10] Cockshott WP. Carpal fusions. Am J Roentgenol 1963;89:1260–71.

[11] Simmons BP, McKenzie WD. Symptomatic carpal coalition. J Hand Surg [Am] 1985;10A(2):190–3.

[12] Poznanski AK, Holt JF. The carpals in congenital malformation syndromes. Am J Roentgenol 1971; 112:443.

[13] Orlin H, Alpert M. Carpal coalition in arthrogryposis multiplex congenita. Br J Radiol 1967;40: 220–2.

[14] Drawbert JP, Stevens DB, Cadle RG, et al. Tarsal and carpal coalition and symphalangism of the Fuhrmann type. J Bone Joint Surg Am 1985; 67A(6):884–9.

[15] Berkowitz AR, Melone CP. Pisiform-hamate coalition with ulnar neuropathy. J Hand Surg [Am] 1992;17A(4):657–62.

[16] Peyton RS, Moore JR. Fracture through a congenital carpal coalition. J Hand Surg [Am] 1994; 19A(3):369–71.

[17] O'Rahilly RA. Survey of carpal and tarsal anomalies. J Bone Joint Surg Am 1953;35A:626–42.

[18] Bogart FB. Variations of the bones of the wrist. Am J Roentgenol 1932;28(5):638–46.

[19] Lane LB, Gould ES, Stein PD, et al. Unilateral osteonecrosis in a patient with bilateral os centrale carpi. J Hand Surg [Am] 1990;15A:751–4.

[20] Yang ZY, Gilula LA, Jonsson K. Os centrale carpi simulating a scaphoid waist fracture. J Hand Surg [Br] 1994;19B(6):754–6.

[21] Poznanski AK, Gall JC, Stern AM. Skeletal manifestations of the Holt-Oram syndrome. Radiology 1970;94:45–53.

[22] Kose N, Ozcelik A, Gunal I. The crowded wrist—a case with accessory carpal bones. Acta Orthop Scand 1999;70(1):96–8.

[23] Adolfsson L. Arthroscopic removal of os centrale carpi causing wrist pain. Arthroscopy 2000;16(5): 537–9.

[24] Koizumi M, Kanda T, Satoh S, et al. Attritional rupture of the flexor digitorum profundus tendon to the index finger caused by accessory carpal bone in the carpal tunnel: a case report. J Hand Surg [Am] 2005;30A:142–6.

[25] Postacchini F, Ippolito E. Isolated absence of human carpal bones. Teratology 1975;11:267–72.

[26] Kuz JE, Smith JM. Congenital absence of the scaphoid without other congenital abnormality: a case report. J Hand Surg [Am] 1997;22A:489–91.

[27] Papanikolaou P, Haddadin MA. Congenital absence of carpal scaphoid. Br Med J 1972;2(808): 292.

[28] Anderson WJ, Bowers WH. Congenital absence of the triquetrum: a case report. J Hand Surg [Am] 1985;10A(5):620–2.

[29] Kao SD, Watson HK, Fong D. Congenital triquetral absence: a case report of an asymptomatic wrist. J Hand Surg [Am] 1996;21(2):314–6.

[30] Treble NJ. Congenital absence of the scaphoid in the "VATER" association. J Hand Surg [Br] 1985;10B(2):251–2.

[31] James MA, McCarroll HR, Manske PR. The spectrum of radial longitudinal deficiency: a modified classification. J Hand Surg [Am] 1999;24: 1145–55.

[32] Bayne LG, Klug MS. Long-term review of the surgical treatment of radial deficiencies. J Hand Surg [Am] 1987;12:169–79.

[33] Havenhill TG, Manske PR, Patel A, et al. Type 0 ulnar longitudinal deficiency. J Hand Surg [Am] 2005;30A:1288–93.

[34] Bayne LG. Ulnar club hand (ulnar deficiencies). In: Green DP, editor. Operative hand surgery. Vol 1. 3rd edition. New York: Churchill Livingstone; 1993. p. 288–303.

[35] Gibson DA, Urs NDK. Arthrogryposis multiplex congenita. J Bone Joint Surg Br 1970;52B(3): 483–93.

[36] Drachman DB, Coulombre AJ. Experimental clubfoot and arthrogryposis multiplex congenita. Lancet 1962;2:523–6.

[37] Drummond DS, Siller TN, Cruess RL. Management of arthrogryposis multiplex congenita. In: AAOS Instructional Course Lectures, Vol 23. St. Louis (MO): CV Mosby Co; 1974. p. 79–95.

[38] Williams PF. Management of upper limb problems in arthrogryposis. Clin Orthop Relat Res 1985;194:60–7.

[39] Bayne LG. Hand assessment and management of arthrogryposis multiplex congenita. Clin Orthop Relat Res 1985;194:68–73.

[40] Bennett JB, Hansen PE, Granberry WM, et al. Surgical management of arthrogryposis in the upper extremity. J Pediatr Orthop 1985;5:281–6.

[41] Wenner SM, Saperia BS. Proximal row carpectomy in arthrogrypotic wrist deformity. J Hand Surg [Am] 1987;12A(4):523–5.

[42] Meyn M, Ruby L. Arthrogryposis of the upper extremity. Orthop Clin N Am 1976;7:501–9.

[43] De Smet AA. Acro-osteolysis occurring in a patient with idiopathic multicentric osteolysis. Skeletal Radiol 1980;5:29–34.

[44] Erickson CM, Hirschberger M, Stickler GB. Carpal-tarsal osteolysis. J Pediatr 1978;93(5):779–82.

[45] Vichi GF, Falcini F, Pierattelli M, et al. Case report 401. Skeletal Radiol 1986;15:665–71.

[46] Beals RK, Bird CB. Carpal and tarsal osteolysis. J Bone Joint Surg Am 1975;57A(5):681–6.

[47] Gluck J, Miller JJ III. Familial osteolysis of the carpal and tarsal bones. J Pediatr 1972;81(3):506–10.

[48] Suri M, Light TR. Carpal and tarsal osteolysis: a case report. Loyola University Chicago Orthopaedic Journal 1999;8:36–41.

[49] Connor JM, Horan FT, Beighton P. Dysplasia epiphysialis hemimelica: a clinical and genetic study. J Bone Joint Surg Br 1983;65B(3):350–4.

[50] Fairbank TJ. Dysplasia epiphysialis hemimelica (tarso-epiphysial aclasis). J Bone Joint Surg Am 1956;38B(1):237–57.

[51] Trevor D. Tarso-epiphysial aclasis: a congenital error of epiphysial development. J Bone Joint Surg Br 1950;32B(2):204–13.

[52] Kettelkamp DB, Campbell CJ, Bonfiglio M. Dysplasia epiphysealis hemimelica: a report of fifteen cases and a review of the literature. J Bone Joint Surg Am 1966;48A(4):746–66.

[53] Lamesch AJ. Dysplasia epiphysealis hemimelica of the carpal bones: report of a case and review of the literature. J Bone Joint Surg Am 1983;65A(3):398–400.

[54] Taniguchi Y, Tamaki T. Dysplasia epiphysealis hemimelica with carpal instability. J Hand Surg [Br] 1998;23B(3):425–7.

[55] Rao SB, Roy DR. Dysplasia epiphysealis hemimelica: upper limb involvement with associated osteochondroma. Clin Orthop Relat Res 1994;307:103–9.

[56] Buckwalter JA, El-Khoury GY, Flatt AE. Dysplasia epiphysealis hemimelica of the ulna. Clin Orthop Relat Res 1978;135:36–8.

[57] Poli G, Verni E. Dysplasia epiphysealis hemimelica of the radius. Chir Organi Mov 1995;80(3):341–4.

[58] Beer TA, Chidgey LK, Wright TW. Dysplasia epiphysealis hemimelica of the carpus. J Surg Orthop Adv 2005;14(1):42–7.

[59] Chinegwundoh JOM, Gupta M, Scott WA. Ulnar dimelia: is it a true duplication of the ulna? J Hand Surg [Br] 1997;22B(1):77–9.

[60] Sandrow RE, Sullivan PD, Steel HH. Hereditary ulnar and fibular dimelia with peculiar facies. J Bone Joint Surg Am 1970;52A(2):367–70.

[61] Laurin CA, Favreau JC, Labelle P. Bilateral absence of the radius and tibia with bilateral reduplication of the ulna and fibula. J Bone Joint Surg Am 1964;46A(1):137–42.

[62] Gorriz G. Ulnar dimelia–a limb without anteroposterior differentiation. J Hand Surg [Am] 1982;7A(5):466–9.

[63] Barton NJ, Buck-Gramcko D, Evans DM. Soft-tissue anatomy of mirror hand. J Hand Surg [Br] 1986;11B(3):307–19.

[64] Gropper PT. Ulnar dimelia. J Hand Surg [Am] 1983;8(4):487–91.

[65] Barton NJ, Buck-Gramcko D, Evans DM, et al. Mirror hand treated by true pollicization. J Hand Surg [Br] 1986;11B(3):320–36.

[66] Harrison RC, Pearson MA. Ulnar dimelia. J Bone Joint Surg Am 1960;42B(3):549–55.

[67] Burgess RC, Cates H. Deformities of the forearm in patients who have multiple cartilaginous exostosis. J Bone Joint Surg Am 1993;75A(1):13–8.

[68] Bock GW, Reed MH. Forearm deformities in multiple cartilaginous exostoses. Skeletal Radiol 1991;20(7):483–6.

[69] Peterson HA. Deformities and problems of the forearm in children with multiple hereditary osteochondromata. J Pediatr Orthop 1994;14:92–100.

[70] Dahl MT. The gradual correction of forearm deformities in multiple hereditary exostoses. Hand Clin 1993;9(4):707–18.

[71] Pritchett JW. Lengthening of the ulna in patients with hereditary multiple exostoses. J Bone Joint Surg Br 1986;68B:561–5.

[72] Tetsworth K, Krome J, Paley D. Lengthening and deformity correction of the upper extremity by the Ilizarov technique. Orthop Clin N Am 1991;22:689–713.

[73] Wood VE, Sauser D, Mudge D. The treatment of hereditary multiple exostosis of the upper extremity. J Hand Surg [Am] 1985;10A:505–13.

[74] Siffert RS, Levy RN. Correction of wrist deformity in diaphyseal aclasia by stapling. J Bone Joint Surg Am 1965;47A:1378–80.

[75] Houshian S, Schroder HA, Weeth R. Corrrection of Madelung's deformity by the Ilizarov technique. J Bone Joint Surg Br 2004;86B:536–40.

[76] Henry A, Thorburn MJ. Madelung's deformity: a clinical and cytogenetic study. J Bone Joint Surg Br 1967;49B:66–73.

[77] Vickers D, Nielsen G. Madelung deformity: surgical prophylaxis (physiolysis) during the late growth period by resection of the dyschondrosteosis lesion. J Hand Surg [Br] 1992;17B:401–7.

[78] Carter PR, Ezaki M. Madelung's deformity: surgical correction through the anterior approach. Hand Clin 2000;16(4):713–21.

[79] Salon A, Serra M, Pouliquen JC. Long-term follow-up of surgical correction of Madelung's deformity with conservation of the distal radioulnar joint in teenagers. J Hand Surg [Br] 2000;25B(1): 22–5.

[80] Lamberti PM, Light TR. Carpal tunnel syndrome in children. Hand Clin 2002;18:331–7.

[81] Light TR. Carpal injuries in children. Hand Clin 2000;16(4):513–22.

[82] Cook PA, Yu JS, Wiand W, et al. Suspected scaphoid fractures in skeletally immature patients: application of MRI. J Comput Assist Tomogr 1997; 21(4):511–5.

[83] Vahvanen V, Westerlund M. Fracture of the carpal scaphoid in children. Acta Orthop Scand 1980;51: 909–13.

[84] Cockshott WP. Distal avulsion fractures of the scaphoid. Br J Radiol 1980;53:1037–40.

[85] Albert MC, Barre PS. A scaphoid fracture associated with a displaced distal radial fracture in a child. Clin Orthop Relat Res 1989;240:232–5.

[86] Christodoulou AG, Colton CL. Scaphoid fractures in children. J Pediatr Orthop 1986;6:37–9.

[87] Mintzer C, Waters PM. Acute open reduction of a displaced scaphoid fracture in a child. J Hand Surg [Am] 1994;19A(5):760–1.

[88] Stanciu C, Dumont A. Changing patterns of scaphoid fractures in adolescents. Can J Surg 1994;37: 214–6.

[89] Suzuki K, Herbert TJ. Spontaneous correction of dorsal intercalated segment instability deformity with scaphoid malunion in the skeletally immature. J Hand Surg [Am] 1993;18A:1012–5.

[90] Anderson WJ. Simultaneous fracture of the scaphoid and capitate in a child. J Hand Surg [Am] 1987; 12A:271–3.

[91] Compson JP. Trans-carpal injuries associated with distal radial fractures in children: a series of three cases. J Hand Surg [Br] 1992;17B: 311–4.

[92] Mazur K, Stevanovic M, Schnall SB, et al. Scaphocapitate syndrome in a child associated with a distal radius and ulna fracture. J Orthop Trauma 1997; 11(3):230–2.

[93] Kamano M, Fukushima K, Honda Y. Multiple carpal bone fractures in an eleven-year-old. J Orthop Trauma 1998;12(6):445–8.

[94] Young TB. Isolated fracture of the capitate in a 10-year-old boy. Injury 1986;17(2):133–4.

[95] Khan SJ, Sherry DD. Kienbock's disease–avascular necrosis of the carpal lunate bone in a 7-year-

[96] Rasmussen F, Schantz K. Lunatomalacia in a child. Acta Orthop Scand 1987;58(1):82–4.

[97] Edelson G, Reis ND, Fuchs D. Recurrence of Kienbock disease in a twelve-year-old after radial shortening. Report of a case. J Bone Joint Surg Am 1988;70:1243–5.

[98] Foster RJ. Kienbock's disease in an 8-year-old girl: a case report. J Hand Surg [Am] 1996;21A(4): 595–8.

[99] Yasuda M, Okuda H, Egi T, et al. Temporary scapho-trapezoidal joint fixation for Kienbock's disease in a 12-year-old girl: a case report. J Hand Surg [Am] 1998;23A:411–4.

[100] Ferlic DC, Morin P. Idiopathic avascular necrosis of the scaphoid: Preiser's disease? J Hand Surg [Am] 1989;14A:13–6.

[101] Preiser G. Eine typische posttraummatische und zur spontanfraktur fuhrende ostitis des naviculare carpi. Fortschur Geb Roentgenstrahlen 1910; 15(4):189–97.

[102] Aptekar RG, Klippel JH, Becker KE, et al. Avascular necrosis of the talus, scaphoid, and metatarsal head in systemic lupus erythematosus. Clin Orthop Relat Res 1974;101:127–8.

[103] Harper PG, Trask C, Souhami RL. Avascular necrosis of bone caused by combination chemotherapy without corticosteroids. Br Med J (Clin Res Ed) 1984;288:267–8.

[104] Kawai H, Tsuyuguchi Y, Yonenobu K, et al. Avascular necrosis of the carpal scaphoid associated with progressive systemic sclerosis. Hand 1983; 15(3):270–3.

[105] Milgram JW, Riley LH. Steroid-induced avascular necrosis of bones in 18 sites: a case report. Bull Hosp Joint Dis 1976;37(1):11–23.

[106] Zadeh HG, Sakka SA, MacLellan GE. Idiopathic avascular necrosis of the scaphoid–a case of early diagnosis by MRI. Acta Orthop Scand 1996; 67(3):298–300.

[107] Ekerot L, Eiken O. Idiopathic avascular necrosis of the scaphoid. Scand J Plast Reconstr Surg Hand Surg 1981;15:69–72.

[108] Allen PR. Idiopathic avascular necrosis of the scaphoid. J Bone Joint Surg Am 1983;65B(3): 333–5.

[109] Herbert TJ, Lanzetta M. Idiopathic avascular necrosis of the scaphoid. J Hand Surg [Br] 1993; 19B:174–82.

[110] Light TR. Injury to the immature carpus. Hand Clin 1988;4(3):415–24.

[111] Laxer RM, Clarke HM. Rheumatic disorders of the hand and wrist in childhood and adolescence. Hand Clin 2000;16(4):659–71.

[112] Chaplin D, Pulkki T, Saarimaa A, et al. Wrist and finger deformities in juvenile rheumatoid arthritis. Acta Rheumatol Scand 1969;15:206–23.

[113] Weinberger A, Ansell BM, Evans D. Wrist involvement in juvenile chronic arthritis five years after onset of disease. Isr J Med Sci 1982;18(5):653–4.

[114] Evans DM, Ansell BM, Hall MA. The wrist in juvenile arthritis. J Hand Surg [Am] 1991;16B(3):293–304.

[115] Jay S, Helm S, Wray BB. Juvenile rheumatoid arthritis. Am Fam Physician 1982;26(2):139–47.

[116] Harel L, Wagner-Weiner L, Poznanski AK, et al. Effects of methotrexate on radiologic progression in juvenile rheumatoid arthritis. Arthritis Rheum 1993;36(10):1370–4.

[117] Granberry WM, Brewer EJ. Results of synovectomy in children with rheumatoid arthritis. Clin Orthop Relat Res 1974;101:120–6.

[118] Rosenberg AM. Uveitis associated with childhood rheumatic diseases. Curr Opin Rheumatol 2002; 14(5):542–7.

ELSEVIER
SAUNDERS

Hand Clin 22 (2006) 465–473

HAND
CLINICS

Kienböck's Disease: An Approach to Treatment

Jeffrey Luo, MD, Edward Diao, MD*

*Division of Hand, Upper Extremity, and Microvascular Surgery, Department of Orthopaedic Surgery,
University of California San Francisco, 500 Parnassus Avenue, MU-320W, San Francisco, CA 94143, USA*

In 1910, Robert Kienböck published his seminal article on traumatic malacia of the lunate [1,2]. Kienböck, a Viennese radiologist, presented radiographic evidence of changes in the proximal portion of the lunate and the radiolunate articulation [3]. He described collapse of the lunate, and believed the cause to be "disturbance in the nutrition of the lunate caused by the rupture of the ligaments and blood vessels during contusions, sprains, or subluxations." He recommended symptomatic treatment, with excision of the lunate reserved for advanced cases.

Kienböck's disease is a clinical condition of the wrist joint characterized by pain over the dorsum of the wrist accompanied by limited wrist motion [4]. There is no gender preference, although patients tend to be younger [5–7]. Symptoms may be present for months to years before patients seek medical attention. More precisely, patients in the early stages of the disease rarely seek treatment; this creates difficulties in knowing the true incidence and the natural history of the disease. Unfortunately, the most advanced form of the condition results in lunate fragmentation with collapse, osteoarthritic changes in the radiocarpal and midcarpal joints caused by the secondary involvement of the surrounding carpal bones, and severe pain. Because of an incomplete understanding of the disease, Kienböck's remains a challenging clinical problem for both the physician and the patient.

Etiology

The etiology of Kienböck's disease remains controversial. Many theories have been proposed; the most common are related to local vascular or osseous anatomy. Although the ultimate pathogenesis may in fact be a complex interplay of different factors, the authors will briefly discuss some of the most prevalent ideas.

Kienböck originally believed the cause to be a disturbance in the nutrition to the lunate. As such, much work has examined the patterns of lunate blood supply and osteonecrosis. There are multiple patterns of arterial supply, with the lunate receiving nutrient vessels from both a volar and dorsal capsular plexus [8]. Further studies revealed that the lunate was supplied by a single palmar artery in 7% of wrists, and that 31% of specimens showed a single path of the artery through bone without significant arborization [9]. A lunate with a single vessel or minimal branching may be at increased risk of osteonecrosis; however, reports of severe injury to the carpus, such as with lunate and perilunate dislocations, often have no or only transient osteonecrosis of the lunate [10]. This may be because the lunate dislocates palmarly, allowing a flap of the palmar capsule with the volar artery to remain intact.

Disruption of the venous outflow, akin to avascular necrosis of the femoral head, has also been suggested as a cause of Kienböck's disease. Shiltenwolf and colleagues [11] reported significantly higher intraosseous pressures with wrist extension in necrotic lunates as compared with normal lunates and control capitates. Unfortunately, it is unclear whether the impaired venous drainage is a cause or a result of the disease, or perhaps a secondary effect of the collapsed bone.

Local osseous anatomy may play an important role in the development of Kienböck's disease. In 1928, Hultén [12] found that negative ulnar variance was present in 78% of his patients who had Kienböck's disease, as compared with 23% in the general population. Hultén suggested that

---

* Corresponding author.
E-mail address: diaoe@orthosurg.ucsf.edu (E. Diao).

0749-0712/06/$ - see front matter © 2006 Elsevier Inc. All rights reserved.
doi:10.1016/j.hcl.2006.07.003

a short distal ulna increased the force transmission across the radiolunate joint, contributing to the increased risk of osteonecrosis. One further study has supported these data [13], whereas others found no statistically significant difference in ulnar variance between patients who had Kienböck's disease and normal controls [14–16]. Kristensen and coworkers [14] described subchondral bone formation in the distal radius in patients at long-term follow-up (mean 20.5 years), leading to the appearance of ulnar negative variance. Both D'Hoore and colleagues [16] and Nakamura and coworkers [17], though finding no relationship between variance and presence of disease, did find a correlation between variance and age. Bonzar and colleagues [18] readdressed this issue by eliminating the confounding variable of age. They confirmed that increasing age was correlated with increasingly positive ulnar variance, as well as the presence of Kienböck's disease. Their study confirmed the association between ulnar variance and Kienböck's disease, independent of age. Unfortunately, causation cannot be inferred from association. Therefore, the link between ulnar variance and Kienböck's disease remains unclear. It is always possible that ulnar variance may simply be a marker for other developmental anomalies that lead to Kienböck's disease.

Decreased radial inclination may also lead to Kienböck's disease [19–21]. Furthermore, anatomic studies [19,21] have suggested that a change in the geometry of the lunate itself, specifically a smaller lunate, may be associated with the disease state. These studies show that changes in radial inclination and in the geometry of the lunate may also play contributory roles in the development of Kienböck's disease. In combination with either isolated or repetitive trauma, an anomaly in vascular or osseous anatomy may predispose the patient to osteonecrosis of the lunate.

Finally, mention should be made of the case reports of Kienböck's disease in association with various systemic diseases, including corticosteroid use [22], sickle cell disease [23], and cerebral palsy [24,25]. There is no unifying theory for pathogenesis, nor is there any evidence that screening for Kienböck's disease is indicated in any of these conditions.

Diagnosis and staging

Kienböck's disease affects patients of all ages and either gender. There need not be a history of antecedent trauma or previous wrist problems.

Symptoms tend to reflect the severity of the disease, ranging from mild discomfort to debilitating pain; however, this is not always the case, because some patients who have radiographic evidence of severe arthrosis remain relatively asymptomatic. Swelling and synovitis is commonly found about the lunate, both on the dorsal as well as the volar side. Wrist range of motion is often reduced, as is grip strength.

In 1977, Lichtman [6] proposed a staging system that described the clinical and radiologic classification for Kienböck's disease (Table 1). This system is now routinely used to stage the disease, guide treatment, and compare outcomes. There have been subsequent modifications to allow for the use of newer technologies, including MRI.

In Stage I, patients present with nonspecific pain suggestive of a wrist sprain or synovitis. Plain radiographs are either normal or demonstrate only a linear fracture of the lunate, with no sclerosis or collapse. MRI is ideal for this early stage, because the uniformly decreased signal intensity of both T1- and T2-weighted images in comparison with the neighboring bones reflects the loss of vascularity. Other causes of T1 signal loss must be considered in the differential diagnosis, including ulnar abutment, lunate fracture, and tumor. Furthermore, increased T2 signal intensity may represent revascularization. This finding is especially valuable in assessing lunate healing during and after treatment.

Lunate sclerosis is the hallmark of Stage II. One or more fracture lines may be present. Significantly, there is no loss of lunate height or other carpal involvement. Patients often present with chronic synovitis.

Table 1
Lichtman's classification of Kienböck's disease

Stage I	Normal radiographs or linear fracture. On MRI, lunate shows low signal on T1-weighted images, and low or high intensity on T2-weighted images.
Stage II	Lunate sclerosis on radiographs. Fracture lines may be present.
Stage IIIa	Lunate collapse, with normal carpal alignment and height
Stage IIIb	Lunate collapse, with decreased carpal height, proximal migration of capitate, and fixed scaphoid flexion (ring sign)
Stage IV	Lunate collapse with peri-lunate degenerative changes

In Stage III, the lunate collapses. This stage is further divided into two categories. In Stage IIIa, carpal height is maintained. Stage IIIb is characterized by proximal migration of the capitate. Also, fixed hyperflexion of the scaphoid leads to the "ring sign." Stage IV heralds the onset of radiocarpal or midcarpal arthritis. These patients typically describe progressive wrist stiffness and symptoms consistent with their degenerative changes.

Natural history

The value of any staging system of a clinical condition lies in its ability to guide treatment; however, mention should be made first of the natural history of the disease. In short, the natural history of Kienböck's disease is not known. Because of the difficulty of performing a definitive study to answer questions about this, few studies have been undertaken, each with low numbers and systematic flaws that the authors acknowledged [5,26]. No prospective data have yet been obtained. Keith and colleagues [5] concluded that Kienböck's disease is a progressive disease that ends in Stage IV changes, despite acknowledging that multiple patients had not progressed beyond Stage IIIa on final follow-up. In contrast, Kristensen and coworkers [26] felt that Kienböck's disease had a "naturally benign course." A few studies have compared untreated patients to different surgical interventions [6,7,27,28], allowing for indirect examination of the natural history by examining the subset of patients without surgical intervention. Taking into account the nonrandomized nature of these studies, there is some suggestion that patients who do not receive surgical treatment do well, but possibly not as well as with surgery. Eaton, however, has collected several patients in the Lichtman Stage IIIb and IV categories who received no treatment beyond a short period of cast immobilization. These patients subsequently revascularized to display normal carpal height and normal lunate shape on follow-up radiographs (personal communication).

Treatment

The combination of unknown etiology and unknown natural history has led to a large, and sometimes baffling, array of surgical procedures that are difficult to compare.

Because of the many surgical options, the authors will first discuss the different procedures based on their underlying principles in regard to how they attempt to remedy the pathogenesis of the disease. Then we will discuss our approach to treatment of patients who have Kienböck's disease.

Surgical treatment strategies fall into three main categories: biomechanical unloading of the lunate, vascularized bone graft, and salvage. Previous generations of patients were treated with prolonged immobilization [6,29] based on Stahl's early reports that 50% of patients were improved or cured after at least two months in a plaster cast [30]. Casting as a primary treatment for symptomatic Kienböck's disease is no longer considered sufficient [6], but short-term immobilization may lessen synovitis and improve symptoms by reducing loads across the lunate. There may be some cases in which cast treatment alone may be sufficient to ameliorate symptoms and affect the natural history of the disease, but this has not been demonstrated in a controlled study.

Joint-leveling procedures are one way to unload the lunate. These procedures are focused on alteration of the bony anatomy in patients who have negative ulnar variance. They include radial shortening osteotomies and the uncommonly performed ulnar lengthening procedures [31,32]. Ulnar lengthening requires use of structural iliac crest bone graft, necessitating healing of two osteotomy sites rather than one after a shortening procedure. Horii and coworkers [33] used a simplified two-dimensional wrist model to assess the extent of unloading of the radiolunate joint after various osteotomies. They found that shortening the radius or lengthening the ulna by 4 mm resulted in a 45% decrease in radiolunate load, with only moderate changes at the midcarpal and radioscaphoid articulations. This led to radial shortening as primary treatment for Kienböck's disease [28,34]. These studies reported predictable improvements in pain, grip strength, and range of motion. Unfortunately, there was no improvement in the appearance of the lunate on postoperative radiographs.

Radial wedge or dome osteotomies have also been used for the treatment of Kienböck's disease [17,35]. Unlike radial shortening, use of a wedge or a dome osteotomy to reduce the inclination angle of the distal radius can be applied in patients who have ulnar neutral or ulnar positive variance as well as negative ulnar variance [35]. There is evidence that the osteotomy decreases force across the capitolunate and radiolunate joints [20], as well as increases the contact area between the radius and lunate [36]. At a minimum of 10 year follow-up, Koh and colleagues [37] reported that patients maintained their improvements in pain, grip strength, and range of motion. Osteoarthritic changes were seen in 54% of patients at 5 years, and 73% of patients at 10 years, suggesting again that radiologic progression of the disease persisted despite surgical treatment.

Another strategy to unload the lunate is to perform selective carpal fusions. These include capitohamate (CH) fusions, with and without capitate shortening, and scaphotrapeziotrapezoid fusions (STT) or scaphocapitate (SC) fusions. Biomechanical studies have suggested that capitohamate fusions without shortening do not reduce forces across the radiolunate joint [38,39], although patients do experience decreased pain and improved motion [40]. Capitate shortening with capitohamate fusion has also been described with good clinical results [41]. Biomechanically, Viola and coworkers [42] showed that capitate shortening with capitohamate fusion decreased radiolunate pressure while increasing radioscaphoid pressure, with little effect on mean radiocarpal pressure. The authors have little experience with this technique, and have concerns with possibly causing circulatory compromise in an adjacent carpal bone.

More commonly, STT and SC fusions have been described as a means to successfully reduce load across the lunate by transferring load to the scaphocapitate and radioscaphoid joints [38,39]. Unfortunately, STT arthrodesis also leads to a decrease in wrist range of motion [38]. Several clinical studies have reported decreased pain and increased grip strength on short- and long-term follow-up [43–45], although some of these same studies suggest increased risk of radioscaphoid arthrosis [44,45].

An interesting development is the use of temporary fixation of joints to help unload the lunate, either with an external fixator or temporary STT or SC pinning [46–48]. Yajima and colleagues [46] felt that the STT fusion was important during lunate revascularization, but unnecessary following remodeling of the lunate. Although this technique has been used in isolation [49,50], it is more commonly used in conjunction with a vascularized bone graft [51,52].

Pedicled vascularized bone grafts (VBG) allow implantation of viable osteoclasts and osteoblasts into the abnormal lunate while preserving the native circulation. This allows for primary bone healing with accelerated creeping substitution and new bone formation. Many different VBGs have been described for the treatment of Kienböck's

disease, including use of the pisiform, distal radius, and metacarpals [53–56]. The original description of a vascular pedicle used the second dorsal intermetacarpal artery and vein implanted into bone [47,57]. The more popular techniques currently allow harvesting of a vascular pedicle with bone graft, and include the 4 + 5 extensor compartmental artery (ECA) and the 2,3 intercompartmental supraretinacular artery (ICSRA) [51,52,56]. Both of these VBGs have adequate pedicle length for rotation to the lunate, supply cortical and cancellous bone, and can maintain viability of the bone. Moran and coworkers [52] reported improvement of pain, grip strength, and range of motion following 26 cases of 4 + 5 ECA. Furthermore, they that noted 77% of postsurgical patients did not have radiologic progression or collapse.

Revascularization with a pedicled bone graft can be used as an adjunct, or an alternative, to any of the unloading-type treatments previously discussed. It is especially attractive in patients who have ulnar neutral or ulnar positive variance, which would preclude consideration of radial shortening procedures. As mentioned, it is typically performed with external fixation or temporary pinning of the STT or SC joints to unload the lunate during revascularization.

Table 2
Options for treatment of Kienböck's disease based on staging

Kienböck's stage	Treatment options
Stage I	Immobilization
	Arthroscopy
Stage II and IIIa	Arthroscopy
	Radial shortening osteotomy (with neutral or negative ulnar variance)
	Vascularized bone graft
	Temporary SC or STT pinning
	Radial wedge or dome osteotomy
	Capitate shortening, with or without CH fusion
	Combinations of above treatments
Stage IIIb	STT or SC fusion with or without lunate excision
	Radial shortening osteotomy
	Vascularized bone graft
Stage IV	Proximal row carpectomy
	Wrist fusion
	Wrist arthroplasty
	Denervation

Mention should be made of the possibility that these solutions that are based on biomechanical alterations may also have an important biologic effect. For example, osteotomies may work by stimulating a vascular and inflammatory response, and not just by altering radiocarpal loading. Revascularization of an abnormal lunate may be hastened by the act of surgery as well as the postoperative immobilization and therapy.

With lunate collapse (IIIA, IIIB0), some authors have continued to recommend the above procedures, with variable results [34,44,52,58]. More predictably, lunate excision can be performed with SC or STT arthrodesis if the radioscaphoid joint is well-preserved [59]. With degenerative changes throughout the carpus come different considerations for treatment. It is generally agreed that there is no point in revascularization or attempting to change the biomechanics and load across the lunate. Treatment options are directed toward the pancarpal arthritis, and include proximal row carpectomy, total wrist

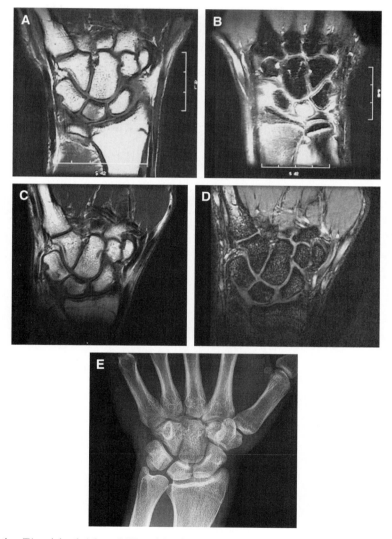

Fig. 1. Preoperative T1-weighted (A) and T2-weighted (B) MRI of a 15-year-old male with Stage I disease and symptoms for over 12 months. (C,D) Repeat MRI 4 months after arthroscopic debridement. There is evidence of revascularization of the lunate. (E) Radiographs 6 months after surgery show no lunate sclerosis. Of note, the patient was ulnar positive, precluding use of a radial shortening procedure.

fusion, and wrist denervation. Even with moderate arthritic involvement of the capitate head and the lunate fossa, a proximal row carpectomy can provide a successful outcome with interposition of dorsal capsule or other material [60,61]. It also helps to preserve an already reduced range of motion, and allows for the possible conversion to total wrist fusion or even a total wrist arthoplasty at a later date. Wrist denervation procedures, although attractive in theory, have not yielded better results than wrist fusion or proximal row carpectomy [62–64]. Of course, wrist denervation can be combined with any of the other procedures to add a measure of symptom-relief in terms of pain control.

Authors' preferred treatment algorithm

The authors' treatment approach is based upon consideration of the natural history of the disease. What is known is that Kienböck's disease exists in diagnosed patients, but the specific natural history in each specific patient is not known. In other words, progression cannot be predicted for an individual patient. Therefore, treatment is predicated on symptom severity and alleviation, with consideration of the stage of disease (Table 2).

Cast treatment can be considered in mildly symptomatic Stage I or II disease, if the patient is willing to undergo temporary immobilization with no guarantee of success. More predictably, wrist arthroscopy can be used in early stage Kienböck's very successfully. Arthroscopy can be used to precisely stage the severity of disease in terms of carpal collapse, cartilage involvement, synovitis, and ligament integrity [65]. The authors have performed arthroscopy on several patients in this stage of disease, based on preoperative symptoms and MRI scans showing changes in lunate signal intensity compared with surrounding carpal bones. The lunates showed mild proximal softening on probe evaluation without loss of cartilage. These patients had synovectomies performed, but no procedures were performed to the bone. Over the next 12 months, symptoms abated, and follow-up MRI scans showed normal lunate signal intensity (Fig. 1).

In more advanced stages of Kienböck's disease, arthroscopy can be used alone or as an adjunct to more traditional open procedures.

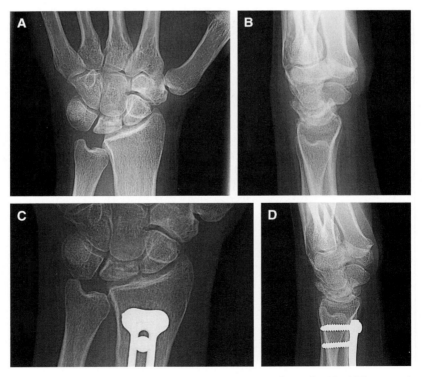

Fig. 2. (*A,B*) 17-year-old female with Stage IIIa disease on preoperative radiographs. (*C,D*) Three months postoperative radiographs with radial shortening and 4 + 5 ECA vascularized bone graft show leveling of the joint.

With more advanced disease, the efficacy of arthroscopy is less predictable; however, the relative ease of recovery from the procedure, and the possibility of treating patients' symptoms with or without supplemental procedures make this surgical option attractive. In these cases, a synovectomy is performed first, followed by inspection of ligaments, all radiocarpal joints and the triangular fibrocartilage complex (TFCC). TFCC tears can be addressed with standard arthroscopic procedures. In cases with moderate chondromalacia, arthroscopic debridement and chondroplasty can be performed. If osteochondral flap tears exist, they can be debrided with a shaver or arthroscopic hand instruments.

In cases of Lichtman Stage IIIb lesions with collapse, arthroscopic evaluation will usually reveal a significantly misshapen and soft proximal lunate. Symptomatic cases are generally best treated by open surgery to excise the lunate, and use of scaphocapitate or scapho-trapezial-trapezoid arthrodesis. Others have advocated radius osteotomy [17,34] and a vascular pedicle procedure [52] for these and claimed satisfactory results (Fig. 2).

For Stage IV disease, salvage procedures are the rule. Proximal row carpectomy can be used, with proximal capitate excision, or with the addition of interposition material, with good success. Alternatively, intercarpal arthrodesis can be considered if the radiocarpal joint is well preserved. Because of lunate involvement, four-corner fusion is not an option. Total wrist arthrodesis, and increasingly, total wrist arthroplasty, complete the treatment options available for severe wrist arthritis, with the indications and results undergoing continual updating. Because recent arthroplasty designs have demonstrated good short-term success, the authors believe they will have an increasing role in these and other complex wrist problems.

Summary

Kienböck's disease remains a difficult entity to treat. Until the etiology and natural history of the disease are understood, treatment will continue to be based on attempts to decrease load across the lunate or bring a blood supply to it. Although these procedures may improve symptoms, it remains unclear whether they will mitigate, halt, or even reverse the natural history of disease progression. For the present, the authors' approach focuses on alleviating patient symptoms, while taking into account the stage of the disease.

References

[1] Kienböck R. Über traumatische Malazie des Mondbeins und ihre Folgezustände: Entartungsformen und Kompressionsfrakturen. Fortschr Roetgenstr 1910;(16):78–103 [in German].

[2] Peltier LF. The classic. Concerning traumatic malacia of the lunate and its consequences: degeneration and compression fractures. Privatdozent Dr. Robert Kienböck. Clin Orthop Relat Res 1980;149:4–8.

[3] Wagner JP, Chung KC. A historical report on Robert Kienböck (1871–1953) and Kienböck's Disease. J Hand Surg [Am] 2005;30(6):1117–21.

[4] Allan CH, Joshi A, Lichtman DM. Kienböck's disease: diagnosis and treatment. J Am Acad Orthop Surg 2001;9(2):128–36.

[5] Keith PP, Nuttall D, Trail I. Long-term outcome of nonsurgically managed Kienböck's disease. J Hand Surg [Am] 2004;29(1):63–7.

[6] Lichtman DM, Mack GR, MacDonald RI, et al. Kienböck's disease: the role of silicone replacement arthroplasty. J Bone Joint Surg Am 1977;59(7):899–908.

[7] Beckenbaugh RD, Shives TC, Dobyns JH, et al. Kienböock's disease: the natural history of Kienböck's disease and consideration of lunate fractures. Clin Orthop Relat Res 1980;149:98–106.

[8] Gelberman RH, Bauman TD, Menon J, et al. The vascularity of the lunate bone and Kienböck's disease. J Hand Surg [Am] 1980;5(3):272–8.

[9] Panagis JS, Gelberman RH, Taleisnik J, et al. The arterial anatomy of the human carpus. Part II: The intraosseous vascularity. J Hand Surg [Am] 1983; 8(4):375–82.

[10] Takami H, Takahashi S, Ando M, et al. Open reduction of chronic lunate and perilunate dislocations. Arch Orthop Trauma Surg 1996;115(2):104–7.

[11] Schiltenwolf M, Martini AK, Mau HC, et al. Further investigations of the intraosseous pressure characteristics in necrotic lunates (Kienböck's disease). J Hand Surg [Am] 1996;21(5):754–8.

[12] Hultén O. Über anatomische Variationen der Handgelenkknochen. Acta Radiol Scand 1928;9: 155–68 [in German].

[13] Gelberman RH, Salamon PB, Jurist JM, et al. Ulnar variance in Kienböck's disease. J Bone Joint Surg Am 1975;57(5):674–6.

[14] Kristensen SS, Thomassen E, Christensen F. Ulnar variance in Kienböck's disease. J Hand Surg [Br] 1986;11(2):258–60.

[15] Nakamura R, Horii E, Imaeda T. Excessive radial shortening in Kienböck's disease. J Hand Surg [Br] 1990;15(1):46–8.

[16] D'Hoore K, De Smet L, Verellen K, et al. Negative ulnar variance is not a risk factor for Kienböck's disease. J Hand Surg [Am] 1994;19(2):229–31.

[17] Nakamura R, Imaeda T, Miura T. Radial shortening for Kienböck's disease: factors affecting the operative result. J Hand Surg [Br] 1990;15(1):40–5.

[18] Bonzar M, Firrell JC, Hainer M, et al. Kienböck disease and negative ulnar variance. J Bone Joint Surg Am 1998;80(8):1154–7.

[19] Tsuge S, Nakamura R. Anatomical risk factors for Kienböck's disease. J Hand Surg [Br] 1993;18(1):70–5.

[20] Watanabe K, Nakamura R, Horii E, et al. Biomechanical analysis of radial wedge osteotomy for the treatment of Kienböock's disease. J Hand Surg [Am] 1993;18(4):686–90.

[21] Thienpont E, Mulier T, Rega F, et al. Radiographic analysis of anatomical risk factors for Kienböck's disease. Acta Orthop Belg 2004;70(5):406–9 [in French].

[22] Culp RW, Schaffer JL, Osterman AL, et al. Kienböck's disease in a patient with Crohn's enteritis treated with corticosteroids. J Hand Surg [Am] 1989;14:294–6.

[23] Lanzer W, Szabo R, Gelberman R. A vascular necrosis of the lunate and sickle cell anemia. A case report. Clin Orthop Relat Res 1984;187:168–71.

[24] De Smet L. Kienböck disease in cerebral palsy. Acta Orthop Belg 2001;67(1):81–3 [in French].

[25] Greene WB. Kienböck disease in a child who has cerebral palsy. A case report. J Bone Joint Surg Am 1996;78(10):1568–73.

[26] Kristensen SS, Thomassen E, Christensen F. Kienböck's disease—late results by non-surgical treatment. A follow-up study. J Hand Surg [Br] 1986;11(3):422–5.

[27] Evans G, Burke FD, Barton NJ. A comparison of conservative treatment and silicone replacement arthroplasty in Kienböock's disease. J Hand Surg [Br] 1986;11(1):98–102.

[28] Salmon J, Stanley JK, Trail IA. Kienböck's disease: conservative management versus radial shortening. J Bone Joint Surg Br 2000;82(6):820–3.

[29] Delaere O, Dury M, Molderez A, et al. Conservative versus operative treatment for Kienböck's disease. A retrospective study. J Hand Surg [Br] 1998;23(1):33–6.

[30] Ståhl F. On lunatomalacia. A clinical and roentgenological study, especially on the pathogenesis and results of immobilization treatment. Acta Chir Scand 1947;95:126.

[31] Roullet J, Walch G. Lengthening technique of the ulna in Kienböck's disease. Results after ten years. Ann Chir Main 1982;1(3):268–72 [in French].

[32] Quenzer DE, Linscheid RL. Ulnar lengthening procedures. Hand Clin 1993;9(3):467–74.

[33] Horii E, Garcia-Elias M, Bishop AT, et al. Effect on force transmission across the carpus in procedures used to treat Kienböck's disease. J Hand Surg [Am] 1990;15(3):393–400.

[34] Weiss AP, Weiland AJ, Moore JR, et al. Radial shortening for Kienböock disease. J Bone Joint Surg Am 1991;73(3):384–91.

[35] Nakamura R, Tsuge S, Watanabe K, et al. Radial wedge osteotomy for Kienböock disease. J Bone Joint Surg Am 1991;73(9):1391–6.

[36] Tsunoda K, Nakamura R, Watanabe K, et al. Changes in carpal alignment following radial osteotomy for Kienböck's disease. J Hand Surg [Br] 1993;18(3):289–93.

[37] Koh S, Nakamura R, Horii E, et al. Surgical outcome of radial osteotomy for Kienböck's disease—minimum 10 years of follow-up. J Hand Surg [Am] 2003;28(6):910–6.

[38] Trumble T, Glisson RR, Seaber AV, et al. A biomechanical comparison of the methods for treating Kienböck's disease. J Hand Surg [Am] 1986;11(1):88–93.

[39] Iwasaki N, Genda E, Barrance PJ, et al. Biomechanical analysis of limited intercarpal fusion for the treatment of Kienböck's disease: a three-dimensional theoretical study. J Orthop Res 1998;16(2):256–63.

[40] Oishi SN, Muzaffar AR, Carter PR. Treatment of Kienböck's disease with capitohamate arthrodesis: pain relief with minimal morbidity. Plast Reconstr Surg 2002;109(4):1293–300.

[41] Almquist EE. Capitate shortening in the treatment of Kienböck's disease. Hand Clin 1993;9(3):505–12.

[42] Viola RW, Kiser PK, Bach AW, et al. Biomechanical analysis of capitate shortening with capitate hamate fusion in the treatment of Kienböck's disease. J Hand Surg [Am] 1998;23(3):395–401.

[43] Watson HK, Ryu J, DiBella A. An approach to Kienböck's disease: triscaphe arthrodesis. J Hand Surg [Am] 1985;10(2):179–87.

[44] Meier R, van Griensven M, Krimmer H. Scaphotrapeziotrapezoid (STT)-arthrodesis in Kienböck's disease. J Hand Surg [Br] 2004;29(6):580–4.

[45] Minami A, Kato H, Suenaga N, et al. Scaphotrapeziotrapezoid fusion: long-term follow-up study. J Orthop Sci 2003;8(3):319–22.

[46] Yajima H, Ono H, Tamai S. Temporary internal fixation of the scaphotrapezio-trapezoidal joint for the treatment of Kienböck's disease: a preliminary study. J Hand Surg [Am] 1998;23(3):402–10.

[47] Tamai S, Yajima H, Ono H. Revascularization procedures in the treatment of Kienböck's disease. Hand Clin 1993;9(3):455–66.

[48] Bochud RC, Buchler U. Kienböck's disease, early stage 3—height reconstruction and core revascularization of the lunate. J Hand Surg [Br] 1994;19(4):466–78.

[49] Yasuda M, Okuda H, Egi T, et al. Temporary scapho-trapezoidal joint fixation for Kienböck's disease in a 12-year-old girl: a case report. J Hand Surg [Am] 1998;23(3):411–4.

[50] Kazuki K, Uemura T, Okada M, et al. Time course of magnetic resonance images in an adolescent patient with Kienböck's disease treated by temporary scaphotrapezoidal joint fixation: a case report. J Hand Surg [Am] 2006;31(1):63–7.

[51] Shin AY, Bishop AT. Pedicled vascularized bone grafts for disorders of the carpus: scaphoid nonunion and Kienböck's disease. J Am Acad Orthop Surg 2002;10(3):210–6.

[52] Moran SL, Cooney WP, Berger RA, et al. The use of the 4 + 5 extensor compartmental vascularized bone graft for the treatment of Kienböck's disease. J Hand Surg [Am] 2005;30(1):50–8.

[53] Kuhlmann JN, Kron C, Boabighi A, et al. Vascularised pisiform bone graft. Indications, technique and long-term results. Acta Orthop Belg 2003;69(4): 311–6 [in French].

[54] Zafra M, Carrasco-Becerra C, Carpintero P. Vascularised bone graft and osteotomy of the radius in Kienböck's disease. Acta Orthop Belg 2005;71(2): 163–8 [in French].

[55] Hurlbut PT, Van Heest AE, Lee KH. A cadaveric anatomic study of radial artery pedicle grafts to the scaphoid and lunate. J Hand Surg [Am] 1997; 22(3):408–12.

[56] Sheetz KK, Bishop AT, Berger RA. The arterial blood supply of the distal radius and ulna and its potential use in vascularized pedicled bone grafts. J Hand Surg [Am] 1995;20(6):902–14.

[57] Hori Y, Tamai S, Okuda H, et al. Blood vessel transplantation to bone. J Hand Surg [Am] 1979;4(1):23–33.

[58] Leblebicioglu G, Doral MN, Atay AA. Open treatment of Sstage III Kienböck's disease with

[59] Takase K, Imakiire A. Lunate excision, capitate osteotomy, and intercarpal arthrodesis for advanced Kienböck disease. Long-term follow-up. J Bone Joint Surg Am 2001;83-A(2):177–83.

[60] Diao E, Andrews A, Beall M. Proximal row carpectomy. Hand Clin 2005;21(4):553–9.

[61] Salomon GD, Eaton RG. Proximal row carpectomy with partial capitate resection. J Hand Surg [Am] 1996;21(1):2–8.

[62] Buck-Gramcko D. Wrist denervation procedures in the treatment of Kienböck's disease. Hand Clin 1993;9(3):517–20.

[63] Linscheid RL. Kienbock's disease. Instr Course Lect 1992;41:45–53.

[64] Foucher G, Da Silva JB, Ferreres A. Total denervation of the wrist. Apropos of 50 cases. Rev Chir Orthop Reparatrice Appar Mot 1992;78(3):186–90 [in French].

[65] Menth-Chiari WA, Poehling GG, Wiesler ER, et al. Arthroscopic debridement for the treatment of Kienböck's disease. Arthroscopy 1999;15(1):12–9.

lunate revascularization compared with arthroscopic treatment without revascularization. Arthroscopy 2003;19(2):117–30.

ELSEVIER
SAUNDERS

HAND
CLINICS

Hand Clin 22 (2006) 475–484

Idiopathic Avascular Necrosis of the Scaphoid: Preiser's Disease

Anthony J. Lauder, MD, Thomas E. Trumble, MD*

*Hand and Microvascular Surgery Program, University of Washington Hand Surgery Institute,
Department of Orthopaedics and Sports Medicine, University of Washington Medical Center,
1959 NE Pacific Street, Seattle, WA 98195, USA*

Idiopathic avascular necrosis of the bones making up the carpus is a relatively rare, albeit often debilitating, condition that most frequently affects the lunate. In 1910, Robert Kienböck [1] initially described a classic case of lunatomalacia, which he believed was caused by vascular compromise. Other carpal bones that can undergo avascular necrosis (AVN) include the capitate [2], pisiform [3], and scaphoid [4]. Since its first description in 1910 [4], Preiser's name has been associated with idiopathic avascular necrosis of the scaphoid. Interestingly, the term idiopathic has probably not been appropriately associated with Preiser because of the fact that all five of the patients that he detailed had a recent history of significant wrist trauma. In fact, a critical reading of Preiser's original work reveals that he was attempting to explain why some scaphoid fractures did not appear until months after the injury. Preiser believed the fractures stemmed from an avascular state that developed after the initial traumatic event. With better plain radiographs and the advantage of CT, it is not unreasonable to believe that Preiser's five patients would have been diagnosed with acute scaphoid fractures. Regardless, although some authors would prefer to define Preiser's disease as post-traumatic AVN of the scaphoid [5], the majority of hand surgeons continue to define Preiser's disease as progressive necrosis of the scaphoid without a known pre-existing fracture.

Although the term Preiser's disease has become synonymous with atraumatic AVN of the scaphoid, many authors have implemented various unique terms to denote the condition. These terms include idiopathic AVN of the scaphoid [5–9], idiopathic osteonecrosis of the scaphoid [10], osteochondritis dissecans of the scaphoid [11,12], and avascular nontraumatic necrosis of the scaphoid [13]. Regardless of the title used to describe the disease, the underlying pathologic process of inadequate blood supply to the scaphoid remains the common denominator. How the scaphoid comes to lose its blood supply remains at a minimum controversial and at best speculative. In 1980 Gelberman and Menon [14] proposed that AVN of the proximal pole of the scaphoid after trauma was likely caused by the pattern of vascularity supplying the scaphoid. In their cadaver study they demonstrated that between 70% and 80% of the proximal scaphoid receives its blood supply from radial artery branches entering through the dorsal ridge (Fig. 1). Waist or proximal pole fractures could most certainly disrupt this single vessel supply to the proximal scaphoid and ultimately lead to AVN. In a follow-up study, Panagis and colleagues [15] grouped the carpal bones into categories based on the size and location of nutrient vessels, the presence of intraosseous anastomoses, and the amount of bone dependent on one nutrient vessel. Group I carpal bones, which included the scaphoid, had large areas dependent on a single vessel with few intraosseous anastomoses. This

* Corresponding author. c/o Tennile N. Monroe, Assistant to Dr. Trumble, Orthopaedics and Sports Medicine, 4245 Roosevelt Way NE, Box 354743, Seattle, WA 98195-4743.

E-mail address: trumble@u.washington.edu (T.E. Trumble).

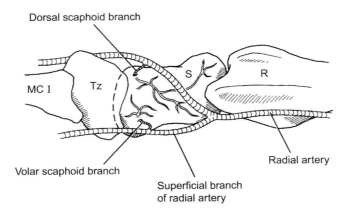

Fig. 1. Illustration of the scaphoid demonstrating that the main blood supply enters on the dorsal and radial aspects. MCI, first metacarpal; R, radius; S, scaphoid; Tz, trapezium. (*From* Trumble TE. Principles of hand surgery and therapy. Philadelphia: W.B. Saunders; 1999. p. 94; with permission.)

group was noted to have a higher incidence of AVN.

Although the term idiopathic infers no antecedent trauma, it is possible that many cases of scaphoid AVN stem from prior injury. Injuries that may have been deemed sprains or simply gone unnoticed could well have been occult scaphoid fractures that ultimately progressed to AVN. It is highly unlikely, however, that every patient who has "idiopathic" osteonecrosis of the scaphoid simply forgot a prior wrist injury or was so immune to the pain stemming from a scaphoid fracture that he did not seek treatment. Further highlighting this point is the fact that more and more cases of scaphoid AVN with no apparent prior trauma are being identified in the literature. To the authors' knowledge there are now at least 57 reported cases of scaphoid osteonecrosis that developed in patients who could not offer any history of wrist injury [5–11,13,16–23].

In an effort to extrapolate a possible etiology for Preiser's disease, several authors have documented conditions and factors associated with AVN of the scaphoid. Several reports have surfaced regarding scaphoid AVN and its possible relationship to chronic steroid usage or systemic collagen vascular disease [22,24–26]. A study by Harper and coworkers [27] detailed the history of a 22-year-old cancer patient who developed multiple sites of AVN (including the scaphoid) after receiving cancer chemotherapy that did not include the administration of systemic steroids. They concluded that combination chemotherapy may induce necrosis of bone even in the absence of steroids. Finally, Kalainov and colleagues [22]

reported on a patient who had a history of "excessive alcohol intake" who developed Preiser's disease. This same patient also had AVN of both femoral heads, a more common site for bony necrosis in alcoholic patients.

Vascular anatomy/biomechanics

Serving as a mechanical link between the proximal and distal carpal rows, the scaphoid is vital for maintaining normal wrist kinematics (the details of which are beyond the scope of this article). To maintain carpal relationships, the scaphoid has five articulations (trapezium, trapezoid, capitate, lunate, and distal radius). Thus, despite its small size, this carpal bone is nearly entirely covered in cartilage (Fig. 2). This correlates with the previously mentioned findings of Gelberman and Menon [14], who found only two perforating vessels entering at ligamentous attachment sites not covered by articular cartilage. A separate study from Taleisnik and Kelly [28] noted three arterial supplies penetrating the scaphoid. They described a distal independent vessel supplying the tuberosity, a lateral-volar vessel supplying the majority of the proximal two thirds of the scaphoid, and a smaller vessel located dorsally and nearer to the proximal pole. After reviewing the results of Taleisnik and Kelly, Gelberman and Menon [14] concluded that the lateral-volar vessel was analogous to the vessel they found entering the dorsal ridge. Importantly, these two studies verify that a single vessel supplies nearly 80% of the scaphoid in a retrograde

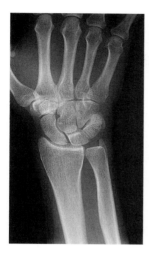

Fig. 2. Plain radiograph demonstrating the five articulations of scaphoid: trapezium, trapezoid, capitate, lunate, and distal radius.

fashion. This vascular anatomy may play a role in the development of Preiser's disease, although no conclusions may yet be drawn.

A 2001 study by Buttermann and colleagues [10] confirmed the presence of a vessel entering the dorsal ridge that supplied the majority of the proximal scaphoid. In addition to further substantiating the tenuous vascular supply of the proximal scaphoid, this study illustrated two other important findings that could feasibly lead to AVN of the scaphoid. First, the authors noted the blood vessel entering through the dorsal ridge had to traverse through a thin intra-articular membrane before penetrating the scaphoid. It was hypothesized that this membrane allowed the scaphoid to rotate, flex, and extend without being tethered to its blood supply. The study authors also postulated, however, that the intra-articular location of the membrane made the vessel susceptible to increased pressures within the joint from such things as effusions or synovitis. This extrinsic pressure, if high enough, could compromise blood flow entering through the dorsal ridge and lead to AVN. The study authors also demonstrated that extrinsic pressure to the vessel entering the dorsal ridge could be exerted by structures outside of the joint. Specifically, they noted that the extensor carpi radialis brevis tendon exerted pressures at the dorsal ridge sufficient to cease blood flow to the proximal scaphoid. This was especially true with the wrist held in 60° or 90° of flexion and 15° of ulnar deviation. Buttermann and colleagues concluded that these new

findings were important factors to consider when delineating conditions that may contribute to idiopathic AVN of the scaphoid [10].

Further supporting the theory that idiopathic osteonecrosis of the scaphoid stems from extra-osseous pathology is the fact that the scaphoid is a load-bearing bone [29,30] with little space to allow penetration of nutrient vessels. Spaces that are available for vessel entrance, areas devoid of hyaline cartilage, are often shared by ligamentous attachments. Importantly, Taleisnik and Kelly [28] noted that some vessels feeding into the scaphoid followed paths in line with carpal ligaments. Based on these findings, many authors have speculated that injury and repetitive micro-trauma to surrounding wrist structures may lead to vascular disruption and Preiser's disease in susceptible patients [5,6,8,10–12,23]. In fact, Herbert and Lanzetta [8] hypothesize that a certain percentage of patients must receive some blood supply through the scapholunate ligament (SLIL) complex (Fig. 3). From clinical observations, these authors noted "numerous" cases in which proximal pole fragments remain viable when their only remaining attachment is to the SLIL. In contradistinction, the authors also report having patients who had proximal pole necrosis after SLIL disruption [8].

Authors have also investigated wrist loading characteristics, specifically ulnar variance, and its relationship to Preiser's disease (Fig. 4). Herbert and Lanzetta [8] noted that seven out of eight of their patients who had idiopathic avascular necrosis of the scaphoid had ulnar positive variance, whereas studies by Kalainov and colleagues [22], Vidal and coworkers [31], and De Smet [13] found no relationship between variance and idiopathic osteonecrosis of the scaphoid. It should be noted, however, that from the report by Herbert and Lanzetta [8] it is difficult to ascertain how the radiographs were taken and how variance was measured. Thus, at this time the data remain inconclusive regarding ulnar variance and its effect on scaphoid vascularity.

Classification

Three classification systems have been devised for grading scaphoids afflicted with Preiser's disease [8,22]. The first scheme, derived by Herbert and Lanzetta in 1993 [8], is based on the progression of the disease as seen with plain radiographs. Based on four stages, this system

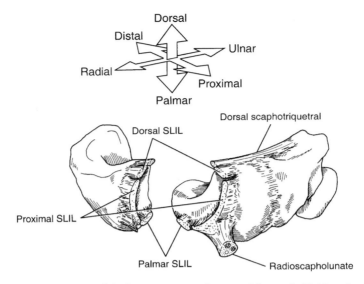

Fig. 3. Illustration demonstrating some of the ligamentous attachments of the scaphoid. Note the three segments of the SLIL, including the strong dorsal portion and the weaker membranous and palmar sections. This ligamentous attachment site may represent an area through which some patients receive blood flow. (*From* Trumble TE. Principles of hand surgery and therapy. Philadelphia: W.B. Saunders; 1999. p. 92; with permission.)

starts at stage 1 with normal radiographs but a positive bone scan, and ends at stage 4 with total collapse of the scaphoid and periscaphoid arthritis (Table 1). Looking at the patient outcomes makes it difficult to derive the prognostic value of this

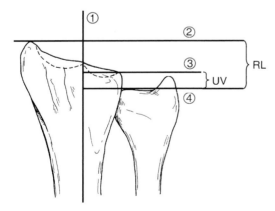

Fig. 4. Ulnar variance is measured as the distance between lines 3 and 4. When the ulna is shorter than the radius it is termed negative ulnar variance. Positive ulnar variance occurs when line 4 is more distal than line 3. RL, relative length of the radius; UV, ulnar variance. (*From* Trumble TE. Principles of hand surgery and therapy. Philadelphia: W.B. Saunders; 1999. p. 130; with permission.)

classification system. Although the study by Herbert and Lanzetta only looked at eight patients, it was interesting to note that two patients who had stage 4 disease fared "Satisfactory" and "Good," whereas one patient who had stage 2/3 disease had only a "Fair" result [8].

Two other systems have been developed, both from the same authors. Kalainov and colleagues [22] described their modified version of the Herbert and Lanzetta system in a 2003 study (Table 2). Ultimately the modifications were relatively minor. These authors implemented another classification scheme based on MRI findings in all 19 of their patients. Individuals were classified as Preiser's type 1 if they had diffuse necrosis of the scaphoid, and as Preiser's type 2 if the necrosis was localized to only a section of the scaphoid

Table 1
Preiser's disease staging as proposed by Herbert and Lanzetta [8]

Stage	Findings (based on plain radiographs)
1	Normal radiographs but positive bone scan
2	Increased proximal pole density plus generalized osteopenia
3	Fragmentation of proximal pole +/− pathologic fracture
4	Carpal collapse with osteoarthritis

Table 2
Modified Herbert and Lanzetta Preiser's disease staging [8] as modified by Kalainov and colleagues [22]

Stage	Findings (based on plain radiographs)
1	Normal radiographs
2	Scaphoid sclerosis, lucencies, and fissuring on plain radiographs
3	Fragmentation of scaphoid
4	Scaphoid collapse and fragmentation with periscaphoid arthritis

(Table 3). Patients who had type 1 necrosis were noted to have higher rates of scaphoid degeneration, lower Mayo wrist scores, and decreased grip strength compared with the patients who had type 2 disease. In addition to better outcome scores, patients who had type 2 necrosis had a higher incidence of reported wrist trauma [22].

Diagnosis

By definition, patients who have Preiser's disease will not have a significant history of wrist trauma or prior scaphoid fracture or surgery; however, patients will frequently relay a history of prior wrist hyperextension or heavy labor. Clinically, the vast majority of patients will present with pain that is insidious and worsening in nature. The pain is often present for months to years before presentation, and it typically localizes to the dorso-radial aspect of the wrist.

On examination, some patients will have mild to moderate swelling over the dorsum or radial aspects of the wrist. This swelling will often worsen with increased loading and use of the wrist. Range of motion and grip strength will generally be reduced, often severely, when compared with the contralateral, presumably normal, wrist. As reported by Kalainov and colleagues [22], the disease occurs approximately two thirds of the time in the dominant wrist. Although Preiser's disease appears to affect adults almost exclusively, there has been one case report of a 10-year-old boy developing fragmentation and necrosis of

the scaphoid with no history of trauma or steroid usage [9].

The radiographic examination should start with four plain radiographs of the wrist, including a zero-rotation posteroanterior (PA), lateral, oblique, and scaphoid (clenched fist PA with ulnar deviation) views (Fig. 5). If the radiographs are normal a bone scan can help localize the problem to the radial carpus; however, a bone scan cannot adequately differentiate between tumors, AVN, or fractures in the scaphoid. Furthermore, after a positive bone scan, patients are often sent for an MRI evaluation, which will not only localize the pathology to the scaphoid but will also define the nature of that pathology. Therefore, the authors avoid bone scans and go straight to an MRI (Fig. 6). A 1990 report by Cristiani and co-workers [32] demonstrated that MRI was very sensitive and more specific than bone scans for AVN of the carpus. The sensitivity and specificity of the MRI can be enhanced by the intravenous injection of gadolinium [33]. CT scans are helpful for defining changes in bony anatomy and are useful adjuncts for preoperative planning.

Treatment

The treatment of idiopathic AVN of the scaphoid remains a confusing and often frustrating dilemma for the treating surgeon. Currently, there is no standardized treatment algorithm for patients affected by Preiser's disease. Because of the lack of treatment protocols many patients are treated conservatively until degeneration of the carpus or pain require that a salvage procedure be performed.

Adding to the confusion from the paucity of treatment guidelines is the number of different

Table 3
Preiser's disease classification as proposed by Kalainov and colleagues [22]

Type	Findings (based on MRI)
1	Diffuse ischemia and necrosis of scaphoid
2	Localized necrosis of scaphoid

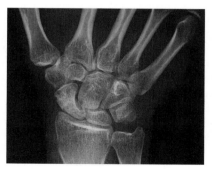

Fig. 5. PA radiograph demonstrating Preiser's disease. Note that this is a true PA with the radial and ulnar styloids making up the far radial and ulnar borders.

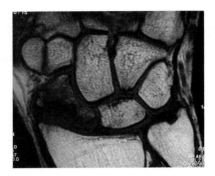

Fig. 6. Coronal section of an MRI demonstrating diffuse necrosis of the scaphoid in a patient with Preiser's disease.

methods reported by various authors for approaching AVN of the scaphoid, each with varying degrees of success. Reported treatments include: (1) splinting [5–8,10,12,22]; (2) proximal row carpectomy (PRC) [12,21,22,34]; (3) proximal scaphoid excision with silastic replacement [7,8]; (4) radial styloidectomy with debridement and bone grafting of the scaphoid [7]; (5) complete scaphoid excision with silastic replacement [7]; (6) total wrist arthroplasty [5]; (7) scaphoid excision with silastic replacement and capito-lunate fusion [5]; (8) scaphoid excision and four-corner fusion [10,22]; (9) scaphoid debridement and vascularized bone grafting [10,22]; (10) scaphoid debridement and cancellous bone grafting [10,22]; (11) debridement of necrotic scaphoid [11]; (12) cortisone injection [22]; (13) electromagnetic bone stimulator [22]; (14) wrist arthrodesis [22]; (15) wrist denervation [7]; and (16) arthroscopic debridement of the scaphoid [23]. Clearly, treatment options of such abundance indicate that an ideal or at least better option has not yet presented itself.

Nonoperative treatments, including observation, anti-inflammatory medications, and splinting, have been reported by many authors [5–10, 21,22,31,34]. Vidal and colleagues [31] treated 5 out of 9 patients with nonoperative measures. Based on the findings that patients treated nonoperatively were only "modestly" limited and those treated surgically were prone to complications, the study authors recommended nonoperative treatment for those who have Preiser's disease. De Smet and coworkers [34] reported their results after treating 2 out of 6 patients by nonoperative means only. One patient had "fair" results, whereas the other patient had no results reported; however, successful nonoperative management has not been demonstrated. The majority of

authors have reported dismal results when nonoperative measures were either initially or definitively chosen as treatment [5–8,10,21,22]. Extrapolating the numbers from these authors [5–8,10,21,22], it is noted that 29 out of 31 patients ultimately failed nonoperative management and had progression of their disease or symptoms. Twenty-six of those 31 patients ultimately went on to require operative treatment for their scaphoid AVN.

The authors' current approach to the patient who has Preiser's disease is a revascularization procedure for those who have necrosis but no degenerative changes and a salvage procedure for those cases that have gone on to arthritic changes. For our revascularization procedures, we prefer to a take a long, narrow graft from the base of the second metacarpal (Fig. 7). The pedicled portion of the graft is based on the dorsal metacarpal arcade that can be found adhering to the bases of the second and third metacarpals. This arcade lies distal to the dorsal intercarpal arch and generally has contributions from both the superficial radial and ulnar arteries [35]. The scaphoid is drilled over its full length from distal to proximal and the graft, shaped much like a matchstick, is then inserted until press-fit into position. Hardware is not required because generally there is no scaphoid fracture to stabilize and the graft is press-fit into the center of the scaphoid. Patients are immobilized with a long-arm thumb spica splint for the initial 10 to 14 days postoperatively. At the first follow-up the splint is converted to a short-arm thumb spica cast, which is generally worn for 2 to 3 months or until signs of graft incorporation are noted (Fig. 8A–D).

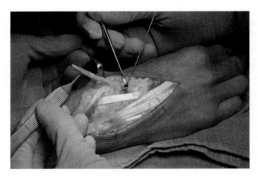

Fig. 7. Intraoperative photograph demonstrating the matchstick-like vascularized graft obtained from the base of the second metacarpal. Forceps are being used to hold the graft. Note the first dorsal compartment crossing over the second dorsal compartment in the proximal portion of the incision.

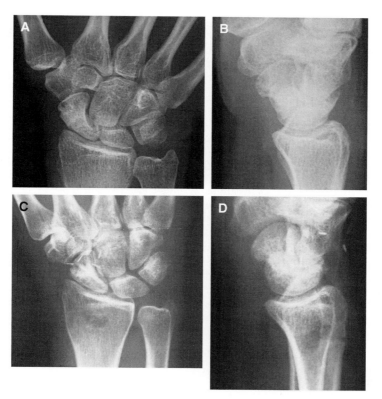

Fig. 8. (*A*, *B*) Preoperative PA and lateral wrist radiographs demonstrating avascular necrosis of the scaphoid with early fragmentation. (*C*, *D*) Postoperative PA and lateral radiographs of the same wrist demonstrating position of the vascularized graft through the longitudinal axis of the scaphoid.

Moran and colleagues [36] recently reported their results of implementing vascularized bone grafts from the distal radius for patients who have scaphoid AVN. Eight patients received vascularized grafts over a 10-year period. Six of the grafts were from the pedicle based off of 1,2 intracompartmental supraretinacular artery, and two of the grafts were based on the 2,3 intracompartmental supraretinacular artery (Fig. 9). Overall, the results were promising and the authors recommended a revascularization procedure for patients who have no fragmentation or degenerative changes of the scaphoid. Seven of the patients had postoperative MRIs, all of which demonstrated evidence of revascularization; however, incomplete revascularization of the proximal pole was a common finding. Motion was relatively maintained and grip strength increased slightly postoperatively. All of the patients reported a reduction in pain. One patient, who initially reported a decrease in pain, ultimately failed revascularization and required a PRC 8 months after the index procedure.

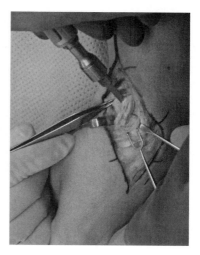

Fig. 9. Intraoperative photograph of a vascularized bone graft bone graft being obtained from the distal radius. The pedicle for this graft was based off of the 1,2 intracompartmental supraretinacular artery. The second dorsal compartment is being retracted toward the bottom of the picture.

After degenerative changes have occurred, a revascularization procedure may correct the AVN of the scaphoid but it will not address the problem of joint loss. Therefore, for advanced cases the authors prefer a salvage type procedure including PRC and scaphoid excision with four-corner fusion (Fig. 10A–F).

Summary

Preiser's disease or idiopathic avascular necrosis of the scaphoid is a rare condition that often presents as vague wrist pain with an insidious onset. At this time an etiology has not been elucidated, but there is evidence to suggest that there may be an anatomical or biomechanical basis for the affliction. In all likelihood the etiology is multifactorial. Patients who are predisposed because of anatomic or biomechanical variations need only another, often relatively minor, insult (minor trauma, steroids, collagen vascular disease) to the blood supply of their scaphoid to compromise the bone's viability.

Several classification schemes have been developed in an effort to help predict prognosis and direct treatment [8,22]. The four stages of Preiser's disease, as described by Herbert and Lanzetta [8], begin with normal plain films but positive bone scan and progress to periscaphoid arthritis. At this time it is difficult to ascertain the prognostic value of this classification system. More recently, Kalainov and colleagues [22] developed a classification system that divides Preiser's disease into scaphoids with diffuse or localized necrosis. In their 2003 study they were able to demonstrate that scaphoids with diffuse (type 1) necrosis were more prone to scaphoid fragmentation and poor outcomes. A diagnosis of Preiser's disease requires scaphoid avascular necrosis with no prior history of scaphoid fracture or surgery. Most commonly the diagnosis can be made with the use of plain radiographs, but one should not hesitate to use MRI for both confirming the diagnosis and evaluating the stage of the disease. Currently, there is no consensus on a proper treatment algorithm. The authors prefer to attempt a revascularization

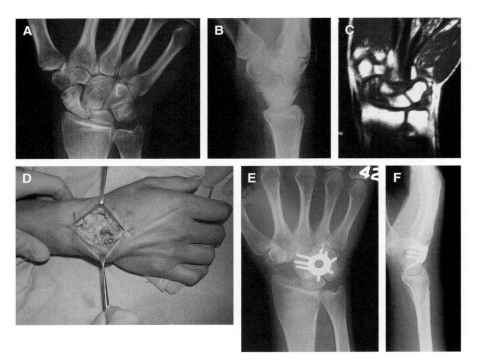

Fig. 10. (A, B) Preoperative radiographs demonstrating Preiser's disease with fragmentation of the scaphoid. (C) Preoperative MRI revealing diffuse necrosis, collapse of the proximal scaphoid, and early degenerative changes. (D) Intraoperative photograph demonstrating a scaphoid excision with four-corner fusion using a Spider Limited Wrist Fusion Plate (Kinetikos Medical Incorporated [KMI], Carlsbad, CA). (E, F) Postoperative radiographs illustrating complete scaphoid excision with early limited wrist fusion.

procedure if the disease is diagnosed early and the scaphoid has not yet gone on to collapse and degenerate, reserving our salvage procedures (four-corner fusion, PRC) for advanced cases with periscaphoid arthritis.

References

[1] Kienböck R. Über traumatische Malazie des Mondbeines und ihre Folgezustände: Entartungsformen und Kompressionsfrakturen [Concerning traumatic malacia of the lunate and its consequences: degeneration and compressions fractures]. Fortschr Geb Roentgenstr 1910–1911;16:77–103 [in German].

[2] Urman JD, Abeles M, Houghton A, et al. Aseptic necrosis presenting as wrist pain in SLE. Arthritis Rheum 1977;20(3):825–8.

[3] Oláh J. Bilaterale aseptische Nekrose des Os pisiforme [Bilateral aseptic necrosis of the os pisiform]. Z Orthop Ihre Grenzgeb 1968;104(4):590–1 [in German].

[4] Preiser G. Zur Eine typische posttraumatische und zur Spontanfraktur führende Ostitis des Naviculare Carpi [A typical fracture leading to spontaneous post-traumatic osteitis of the scaphoid]. Fortschr Geb Roentgenstr 1910;15:189–97 [in German].

[5] Ferlic DC, Morin P. Idiopathic avascular necrosis of the scaphoid: Preiser's disease? J Hand Surg [Am] 1989;14(1):13–6.

[6] Allen PR. Idiopathic avascular necrosis of the scaphoid: a report of two cases. J Bone Joint Surg [Br] 1983;65(3):333–5.

[7] Ekerot L, Eiken O. Idiopathic avascular necrosis of the scaphoid: case report. Scand J Plast Reconstr Surg 1981;15:69–72.

[8] Herbert TJ, Lanzetta M. Idiopathic avascular necrosis of the scaphoid. J Hand Surg [Br] 1993;19:174–82.

[9] Jensen CH, Leicht P. Idiopathic avascular necrosis of the scaphoid in a child: case report. Scand J Plast Reconstr Hand Surg 1995;29:359–60.

[10] Buttermann GR, Putnam MD, Shine JD. Wrist position affects loading of the dorsal scaphoid: possible effect on extrinsic scaphoid blood flow. J Hand Surg [Br] 2001;26(1):34–40.

[11] Guelpa G, Chamay A, Lagier R. Bilateral osteochondritis dissecans of the carpal scaphoid: a radiological and anatomical study of one case. Int Orthop 1980;4(1):25–30.

[12] Cook DA, Engber WD. Osteochondritis dissecans of the scaphoid: Preiser's disease? Orthopedics 1993;16(6):705–7.

[13] De Smet L. Avascular nontraumatic necrosis of the scaphoid: Preiser's disease? Chir Main 2000;19:82–5.

[14] Gelberman RH, Menon J. The vascularity of the scaphoid bone. J Hand Surg [Am] 1980;5(5):508–13.

[15] Panagis JS, Gelberman RH, Taleisnik J, et al. The arterial anatomy of the human carpus. Part II: The intraosseous vascularity. J Hand Surg [Am] 1983; 8(4):375–82.

[16] Alnot JY, Frajman JM, Bocquet L. Primary total aseptic osteonecrosis of the scaphoid bone. Ann Chir Main Memb Super 1990;9:221–5 [in French].

[17] Lenoble E, Mawhinney I. Two unusual cases of avascular necrosis of the scaphoid. Rev Rhum Ed Fr 1994;61:462–5 [in French].

[18] Dossing K, Boe S. Idiopathic avascular necrosis of the scaphoid: case report. Scand J Plast Reconstr Surg 1994;28:155–6.

[19] Martini G, Valenti R, Giovani S, et al. Idiopathic avascular necrosis of the scaphoid: a case report. Recenti Prog Med 1995;86:238–40 [in Italian].

[20] Zadeh HG, Sakka SA, MacLellan GE. Idiopathic avascular necrosis of the scaphoid: a case of early diagnosis by MRI. Acta Orthop Scand 1996;67:298–300.

[21] De Smet L, Aerts P, Fabry G. Avascular necrosis of the scaphoid: report of three cases treated with a proximal row carpectomy. J Hand Surg [Am] 1992;17:907–9.

[22] Kalainov DM, Cohen MS, Hendrix RW, et al. Preiser's disease: identification of two patterns. J Hand Surg [Am] 2003;28(5):767–78.

[23] Menth-Chiari WA, Poehling GG. Preiser's disease: arthroscopic treatment of avascular necrosis of the scaphoid. Arthroscopy 2000;16:208–13.

[24] Dubois EL, Cozen L. Avascular (aseptic) bone necrosis associated with systemic lupus erythematosus. JAMA 1960;174:966–71.

[25] Kawai H, Tsuyuguchi Y, Yonenobu K, et al. Avascular necrosis of the carpal scaphoid associated with progressive systemic sclerosis. Hand 1983;15(3):270–3.

[26] Urman JD, Abeles M, Houghton AN, et al. Aseptic necrosis presenting as wrist pain in SLE. Arthritis Rheum 1977;20(3):825–8.

[27] Harper PG, Trask C, Souhami RL. Avascular necrosis of bone caused by combination chemotherapy without corticosteroids. Br Med J (Clin Res Ed) 1984;288:267–8.

[28] Taleisnik J, Kelly P. The extraosseous and intraosseous blood supply of the scaphoid bone. J Bone Joint Surg [Am] 1966;48:1125–37.

[29] Hara T, Horii E, An K, et al. Force distribution across wrist joint: application of pressure-sensitive conductive rubber. J Hand Surg [Am] 1992;17:339–47.

[30] Kazuki K, Kusunoki M, Shimazu A. Pressure distribution in the radiocarpal joint measured with a densitometer designed for pressure-sensitive film. J Hand Surg [Am] 1991;16:401–8.

[31] Vidal MA, Linscheid RL, Amadio PC, et al. Preiser's disease. Ann Chir Main Memb Super 1991; 10:227–36.

[32] Cristiani G, Cerofolini E, Squarzina PB, et al. Evaluation of ischaemic necrosis of carpal bones by magnetic resonance imaging. J Hand Surg [Br] 1990;15:249–55.

[33] Cerezal L, Abascal F, Canga A, et al. Usefulness of gadolinium-enhanced MR imaging in the evaluation of the vascularity of scaphoid nonunions. AJR Am J Roentgenol 2000;174:141–9.

[34] De Smet L, Aperts P, Walraevens M, et al. Avascular necrosis of the carpal scaphoid: Preiser's disease—report of 6 cases and review of the literature. Acta Orthop Belg 1993;59(2):139–42 [in French].

[35] Sawaizumi T, Nanno M, Nanbu A, et al. Vascularized bone graft from the base of the second metacarpal for refractory nonunion of the scaphoid. J Bone Joint Surg [Br] 2004;86(7):1007–12.

[36] Moran SL, Cooney WP, Shin AY. The use of vascularized grafts from the distal radius for the treatment of Preiser's disease. J Hand Surg [Am] 2006;31(5):705–10.

ELSEVIER
SAUNDERS

Hand Clin 22 (2006) 485–500

HAND
CLINICS

Carpal Dislocations

Ryan J. Grabow, MD[a],*, Louis Catalano III, MD[b]

[a]Nevada Orthopedic & Spine Center, 2650 North Tenaya Way, Suite 301, Las Vegas, NV 89128, USA
[b]C.V. Starr Hand Surgery Center, Saint Luke's-Roosevelt Hospital, 1000 Tenth Avenue, New York, NY 10019, USA

Carpal dislocations are rare injuries. They most often occur from high-energy trauma such as motor vehicle accidents, falls from a height, or industrial-related accidents. Usually occurring in young males in their twenties or thirties, these injuries may be missed initially because of concomitant injuries. A thorough understanding of the carpal anatomy, injury patterns, and treatment options is critical for proper management of these rare but significant injuries. In this article the authors address the five main categories of carpal dislocations, the associated anatomy, and their diagnosis, treatment, and prognosis.

Anatomy

Numerous studies have detailed the complex coordination of movement between the proximal and distal rows of the carpus, and the critical importance of the integrity of the intrinsic and extrinsic ligamentous system to maintain that coordination [1,2]. The extrinsic ligaments that link the radius and ulna to the carpus are divided into three major groups: volar radiocarpal, volar ulnocarpal, and dorsal radiocarpal ligaments.

Volar ligaments

The volar ligaments are the strongest of the extrinsic ligaments, and are the main stabilizers of the radiocarpal joint. There are four volar radiocarpal ligaments: radioscaphocapitate (RSC), long radiolunate (LRL), radioscapholunate (RSL), and short radiolunate (SRL) (Fig. 1). The first three originate from the lateral third of the distal radius on its volar rim. The RSC is the most radial and runs obliquely across the volar waist of the scaphoid to insert on the capitate. It serves as a fulcrum for scaphoid flexion and is the primary restraint to ulnar translocation of the carpus. The LRL is ulnar to the RSC and is a strong tether to lunate displacement. The RSL ligament is felt to be a neurovascular conduit to the scapholunate (SL) ligament, and is not considered a stabilizing structure for the carpus [3]. The SRL ligament is the most ulnar of the radiocarpal ligaments arising from the volar ulnar lip of the distal radius. It travels vertically to insert on the lunate, providing a stabilizing force to prevent dorsal dislocation in hyperextension injuries [3]. The volar ulnar ligaments, which include the ulnocapitate (UC), the ulnotriquetral (UT), and the ulnolunate (UL), link the carpus to the ulna. The UC ligament joins the RSC at the capitate, and together they form the arcuate ligament. Proximal to this point is a capsular weakening called the space of Poirier, through which the capitate or lunate dislocates in complex injuries. The midcarpal joint is stabilized volarly by the scaphotrapeziotrapezoid (STT) ligament, the scaphocapitate (SC), and the triquetrohamatecapitate complex (THC). Also known as the ulnar leg of the distal V or arcuate ligament, the THC is a group of fan-shaped fibers that blend with the UC ligament.

Dorsal ligaments

The two primary dorsal extrinsic ligaments are the dorsal radiocarpal (DRC), also known as the dorsal radiotriquetral, and the dorsal intercarpal ligaments (DIC) (Fig. 2). The DRC extends from the dorsal edge of the radius, centered at Lister's tubercle, and inserts on the triquetrum to control ulnar translation. The DIC extends from the triquetrum to the dorsal distal scaphoid and dorsal

* Corresponding author.
 E-mail address: rgrabowmd@yahoo.com (R.J. Grabow).

0749-0712/06/$ - see front matter © 2006 Elsevier Inc. All rights reserved.
doi:10.1016/j.hcl.2006.07.004

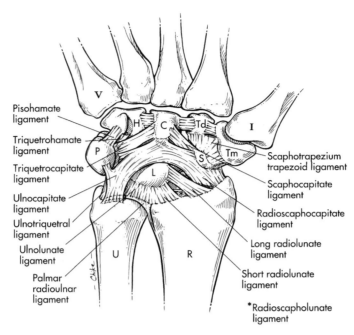

Pisohamate ligament
Triquetrohamate ligament
Triquetrocapitate ligament
Ulnocapitate ligament
Ulnotriquetral ligament
Ulnolunate ligament
Palmar radioulnar ligament

Scaphotrapezium trapezoid ligament
Scaphocapitate ligament
Radioscaphocapitate ligament
Long radiolunate ligament
Short radiolunate ligament
*Radioscapholunate ligament

Fig. 1. Volar carpal ligaments. (*From* Berger RA. Ligament anatomy. In: Cooney WP, Linscheid RL, Dobyns JH, editors. The wrist: diagnosis and operative treatment. St. Louis (MO): Mosby; 1998; with permission.)

aspect of the trapezoid. It provides a dorsal support to translation of the midcarpal joint.

Intrinsic ligaments

The proximal carpal row is an intercalated segment consisting of the scaphoid, lunate, and triquetrum connected via stout interosseous ligaments (Fig. 3). There are no direct tendon insertions on the proximal row; thus the row's kinematics is dependent on the integrity of these ligaments. The SL ligament joins its respective bones and has three separate components: volar, dorsal, and proximal. The dorsal aspect is the

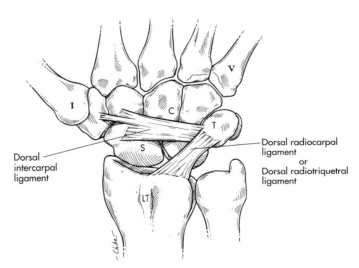

Dorsal intercarpal ligament

Dorsal radiocarpal ligament
or
Dorsal radiotriquetral ligament

Fig. 2. Dorsal carpal ligaments. (*From* Berger RA. Ligament anatomy. In: Cooney WP, Linscheid RL, Dobyns JH, editors. The wrist: diagnosis and operative treatment. St. Louis (MO): Mosby; 1998; with permission.)

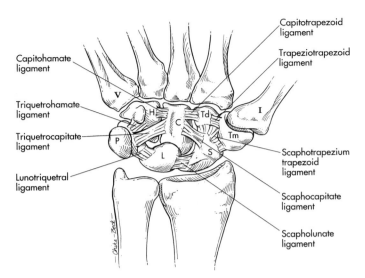

Fig. 3. Intrinsic carpal ligaments. (*From* Berger RA. Ligament anatomy. In: Cooney WP, Linscheid RL, Dobyns JH, editors. The wrist: diagnosis and operative treatment. St. Louis (MO): Mosby; 1998; with permission.)

strongest portion of the ligament and serves to resist excessive scaphoid flexion, translation, and intercarpal supination. The lunotriquetral (LT) ligament, joins the lunate and triquetrum, with its volar portion being the strongest. This ligament is vital to prevent ulnar translation of the triquetrum. The distal carpal row is linked via three primary ligaments: the trapeziotrapezoid (TT), the trapeziocapitate (TC), and the capitohamate (CH) ligaments.

Classification

Carpal dislocations can be divided into five separate groups: (1) perilunate dislocations, or lesser arc injuries; (2) transcarpal fracture-dislocations, or greater arc injuries; (3) radiocarpal dislocations; (4) axial dislocations; and (5) isolated carpal bone dislocations [4].

Diagnosis

Because of the significant force required to overcome the strong ligamentous support of the carpus, there is usually a history of significant high-energy trauma, such as a motor vehicle accident, fall from a height, or industrial accident. In the acute setting, there is obvious pain and swelling of the hand and wrist. Gross deformity of the wrist is usually noted. Often a firm tender mass is noted over dislocated carpal bones. A step-off or void may be

noted in the proximal row if swelling is not yet significant. Most often, deep palpation of the wrist will be intolerable for the patient, and is usually not necessary for diagnosis. On examination the patient may have symptoms of median or ulnar nerve compression caused by swelling or direct impingement by displaced carpal bones. As for all trauma about the wrist, standard posteroanterior (PA) and lateral radiographs should be obtained. Oblique images of the carpus, such as the 45° pronated or supinated views, can give further information and are often helpful in recognition of injuries at the carpometacarpal (CMC) joints. Additionally, PA and lateral views with the carpus in traction can be of great value in defining the full extent of the injury [5]. Advanced imaging with CT or MRI can give further information about the status of the ligamentous injury or fracture pattern when necessary.

Perilunate dislocations

Perilunate dislocations are the most common of the carpal dislocations. Usually occurring in young men in the second or third decade of life, these injuries are the result of wrist hyperextension, often caused by a fall from a height, a motor vehicle accident, or contact sports. The limits of ligamentous and bony constraints are exceeded with palmar tension and dorsal compressive forces of wrist hyperextension. A variety of injury patterns can occur with this mechanism, depending on the position of the extremity at impact, the quality of the bone, the ligamentous strength, and the direction of force [6]. These injuries are rarely seen in the older population, because without good bone quality the distal radius is most likely to fail before the carpal bones or ligaments. In the pediatric population, the hyperextension forces required to cause these injuries usually injure the weaker radial physis rather the carpal ligaments.

Often perilunate dislocations are associated with other concomitant injuries of the bones or soft tissues of the carpus. Carpal fractures or fractures of the radial or ulnar styloid occur more often than purely ligamentous perilunate dislocations. Approximately two thirds of carpal dislocations involve a fracture through the middle third of the scaphoid, with trans-scaphoid perilunate dislocation being the most common injury encountered in all published series [5]. Additionally, a fracture of the capitate is also frequently encountered, present in approximately 8% of all fracture dislocations of the wrist.

Pathomechanics

The concept of a sequential pattern of intercarpal wrist instability was supported by the work of Mayfield and colleagues [6], and resulted in the understanding of perilunate instability as a spectrum of injury they termed "progressive perilunar instability." Divided into four stages, this pattern of injury was reproducible in the laboratory with hyperextension, ulnar deviation, and intercarpal supination of the wrist with an applied axial load. Based on the viscoelastic properties of bones and ligaments, the rate of loading determines the pattern of injury, with slower loading resulting in carpal fractures, and faster loading resulting in ligamentous injury [7].

Classification

Perilunate dislocations are classified based on the bones and joints involved, the direction of displacement, and the degree of rotation of the lunate. Johnson [8] defined pure ligamentous injuries without fracture as "lesser-arc" injuries, and fracture dislocations involving one or more of the carpal bones surrounding the lunate as "greater-arc" injuries (Fig. 4). Most commonly the scaphoid is fractured; however, the radial and ulnar styloids, capitate, and triquetrum can also be involved. Lunate alignment was classified by Witvoet and Allieu [9] based on the degree of angulation. Normal alignment (Grade I), rotated palmarly less than 90° (Grade II), rotated greater

than 90° but still attached by the palmar ligaments to the radius (Grade III), and total enucleation without any soft tissue connections (Grade IV). Although these other classifications are useful to describe fracture patterns and ligamentous disruption, the classification by Mayfield and colleagues [6] is the most commonly used classification system (Fig. 5). The stages of perilunar instability are described as follows.

Stage I: scapholunate dissociation

With forceful distal carpal row extension, supination, and ulnar deviation, the STT and SL ligaments are under tension, resulting in an extension force transmitted to the scaphoid. The scaphoid extends, causing the SL ligament to transmit torque to the lunate. Because of the palmarly located long and short radiolunate ligaments and the UL ligament, the lunate is restricted in its ability to extend, and resists the torque transmitted via the SL ligament. If the extension force to the scaphoid persists, either the scaphoid waist will fracture or the SL ligament will tear from volar to dorsal, eventually resulting in a complete dissociation of the ligament. With this differential extension between the scaphoid and lunate, the space of Poirier is opened.

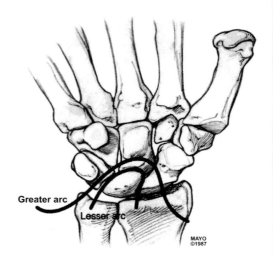

Fig. 4. Greater and lesser arc injuries. Lesser arc injuries are purely ligamentous, whereas greater arc injuries are ligamentous disruptions with associated fractures of the radius, ulna, or adjacent carpal bones. (*From* Tolo ET, Shin AY. Fracture dislocations of the carpus. In: Trumble TE, editor. Hand surgery update 3. Rosemont (IL): ASSH; 2003; with permission.)

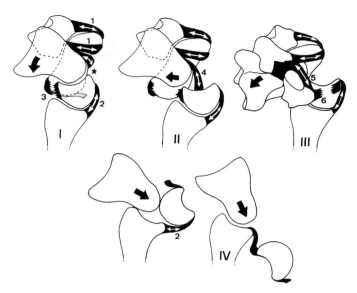

Fig. 5. Progressive perilunate instability. Schematic representation of the four stages of perilunate instability, viewed from the ulnar side. Stage I: As the distal carpal row is forced into hyperextension (*black arrows*), the scapho-trapezio-capitate ligaments (*1*) pull the scaphoid into extension, thus opening the space of Poirier (*asterisk*). The lunate cannot extend as much as the scaphoid, because it is directly constrained by the short RL ligament (*2*). When the SL torque reaches a certain value, the SL ligaments may fail, usually from palmar to dorsal. A complete SLD is`defined by the rupture of the dorsal SL ligament (*3*). Stage II: Once dissociated from the lunate, the scaphoid-distal row complex may dislocate dorsally relative to the lunate (*black arrow*). The limit of such dorsal translation is determined by the RSC ligament (*4*). Stage III: If hyperextension persists, the ulnar limb of the arcuate ligament (*5*) may pull the triquetrum into an abnormal extension, thus causing failure of the lunotriquetral ligaments (*6*). Stage IV: Finally, the capitate may be forced by the still intact RSC ligament (*4*) to edge into the radiocarpal space and push the lunate palmarward until it dislocates into the carpal canal in a rotatory fashion. All white arrows represent the distraction forces occurring in the ligaments. (*From* Garcia-Elias M, Geissler WB. Carpal instability. In: Green DP, Hotchkiss RN, Pederson WC, et al, editors. Operative hand surgery. 5th edition. Philadelphia: Elsevier; 2005. *Modified from* Mayfield JK, Johnson RP, Kilcoyne RK. Carpal dislocations: pathomechanics and progressive perilunar instability. J Hand Surg [Am] 1980;5:2226–41; with permission.)

Stage II: lunocapitate dislocation

As the extension-supination moment continues, the scaphoid-distal row complex is forced into further extension, subsequently leading to a dorsal dislocation of the capitate relative to the lunate over the intact distal edge of the DIC ligament. The capitate is limited in its dorsal displacement by an intact RSC ligament. The entire distal row and the dissociated radial portion of the proximal row follow the capitate dorsally, further opening the space of Poirier.

Stage III: lunotriquetral disruption

After the capitate has dislocated, further extension-supination torque and a dorsal translation vector is transmitted to the triquetrum through the ulnar limb of the arcuate UC ligament. As the triquetrum extends, this torque is transmitted to the LT ligament. If the extension torque continues, a tear of the LT ligament or triquetrum avulsion fracture may result. Usually the LT tear progresses from volar to dorsal. With complete rupture of the LT ligament, the ulnar expansions of the LRL ligament usually also tear, leaving the SRL ligament and the UL ligament as the lunate's only stabilizing forces.

Stage IV: lunate dislocation

If the extension force continues, the dorsally displaced capitate may be pulled proximally and volarly into the radiocarpal space by a still-intact RSC ligament, muscle contraction, or external force. The DRC ligament is disrupted and the capitate pushes the lunate volarly, causing it to hinge on the intact palmar ligaments and displace volarly into the carpal tunnel. Thus, lunate dislocation is the end stage of a dorsal perilunate dislocation.

Diagnosis

Despite continued efforts to educate emergency providers, 16% to 25% of perilunate injuries are initially missed on examination in the emergency department and present late as chronic dislocations [5,10]. A late presentation leads to a significantly poorer outcome and often necessitates a salvage operation. Therefore it is critical for these injuries to be identified acutely. On examination, the patient will have a swollen, tender wrist and pain with minimal range of motion. The neurovascular examination may reveal symptoms of median nerve compression caused by swelling or impingement of the lunate on the carpal tunnel in Stage III and IV dislocations. Standard PA and lateral radiographs may reveal several characteristic findings: (1) foreshortened carpus and loss of carpal height; (2) "triangular-shaped" lunate overlapping the capitate; (3) scaphoid flexion, exhibiting a "ring sign"; (4) a break in Gilula's line proximally between the lunate and triquetrum; (5) prominent dorsal pole of the lunate as it tips into palmar flexion; (6) lunate lying palmar to the radius; and (7) capitate in palmar flexion (Fig. 6).

Treatment

As for any carpal dislocation, the goal of treatment is anatomic reduction of the carpus. In the acute setting treatment should always include closed reduction and immobilization to reduce pressure on the surrounding structures. If closed reduction achieves an anatomic reduction, percutaneous pinning can be combined with immobilization to stabilize the wrist. This was previously the recommended treatment [6]; however, recent literature has shown a high rate of recurrent instability, carpal incongruity, and arthritis. For most injuries, better results have been achieved with open reduction, ligament repair, and internal fixation than with closed methods, and open reduction is now the current standard of care [4–6].

Closed reduction

The technique for closed reduction of a perilunate (Stage I–III) or lunate (Stage IV) dislocation has been described by several authors [11,12]. An essential component is complete muscle relaxation, either through general anesthesia, or Bier's or axillary block. The wrist is then suspended in

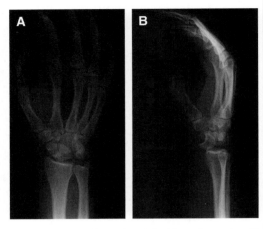

Fig. 6. Injury radiographs: (A) AP radiograph with foreshortened carpus and "triangular-appearing" lunate suggesting abnormal carpal alignment. (B) Lateral radiograph clearly shows palmar flexion of lunate, "spilled teacup" sign, flexion of scaphoid, and capitate collinear with radial shaft in this Stage IV perilunate dislocation, "a volar lunate dislocation."

finger traps with approximately 10 lbs traction for at least 10 minutes to relax muscular spasm. Fluoroscopic assessment of the wrist in traction can be very helpful in assessing the full extent of the injury. After sufficient suspension in traction, the volar distal aspect of the wrist is palpated with the dominant thumb until clearly pressing distally and dorsally on the lunate. While maintaining thumb pressure on the lunate, the finger traps are removed. The wrist is then extended, while the thumb continues to stabilize the lunate. Longitudinal traction is applied manually, and the wrist is slowly flexed while pressing volarly on the lunate. During this maneuver the capitate is brought into flexion and usually reduces onto the lunate with a palpable snap. Maintaining dorsally directed pressure on the lunate during this maneuver is critical to avoid pushing the lunate further volarly. After the capitate has been reduced onto the lunate, the lunate is pushed dorsally while maintaining traction and slowly extending the wrist. The lunate will usually reduce during this maneuver, and full reduction will be achieved (Figs. 7, 8). Fluoroscopy is then used to confirm reduction of the radiolunate and capitolunate joints. The wrist is splinted in neutral position, allowing for motion at the metacarpophalangeal (MCP) joints and digits to help reduce digital swelling and stiffness. Splinting in maximal flexion is not required, and may lead to acute carpal tunnel syndrome. In certain circumstances,

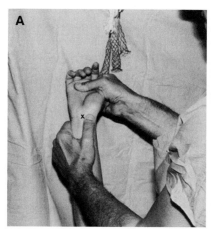
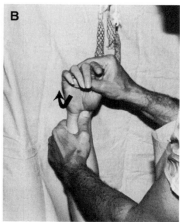

Fig. 7. Perilunate/lunate dislocation closed reduction technique. (*A*) After 10 minutes of uninterrupted traction, and following fluoroscopic traction views of the wrist, the surgeon supports the patient's hand as the finger traps are removed. The wrist is extended and the surgeon places his thumb over the proximal palmar projection of the lunate (*X*). (*B*) While maintaining manual longitudinal traction and applying pressure against the palmar projection of the lunate, the wrist is gradually flexed and the capitolunate reduction is felt as a distinct snap (*arrow*). (*From* Taleisnik J. The wrist. New York: Churchill Livingston; 1985; with permission)

attempts at closed reduction will be ineffective and open reduction will be required. Because of the possible compression of the median nerve caused by a palmarly dislocated lunate, emergent open reduction and subsequent fixation combined

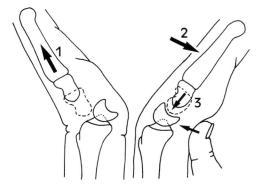

Fig. 8. Schematic representation of the capitolunate reduction based on the original description by Tavernier. (*1*) With the wrist slightly extended, gentle manual traction is applied. (*2*) Without releasing traction, and while the lunate is stabilized palmarly by the surgeon's thumb, the wrist is flexed until a snap occurs. This indicates that the proximal pole of the capitate has overcome the dorsal lip of the lunate. (*3*) Traction is then released and the wrist is brought back into neutral. (*From* Garcia-Elias M, Geissler WB. Carpal instability. In Green DP, Hotchkiss RN, Pederson WC, et al, editors. Operative hand surgery. 5th edition. Philadelphia: Elsevier; 2005; with permission.)

with a carpal tunnel release should be considered if any signs of median nerve compression arise.

Open reduction and repair

Despite the general understanding that surgery provides the best opportunity for a successful outcome, there is still some debate upon the surgical exposure for these injuries. Success has been reported with a dorsal or volar exposure; however, each approach is somewhat limited in providing full access to these carpal injuries. In a multicenter study, Herzberg and colleagues [5] reported that a failure to identify and treat each component of the injury was a major determinant of an unsatisfactory result, and that open reduction and internal fixation achieved better radiographic and clinical results. A combined dorsal-volar approach provides full visualization of the ligamentous and osseous injuries, and enables one to address every aspect of the injury pattern. First reported by Dobyns and Swanson in 1973 [11], the utility of the dual incision approach enables the surgeon to achieve a good outcome. This has been well-supported in the literature, and should most often be employed for injuries Stage II or greater [4,13–15].

Reduction of the lunate to the radius, reduction of the scaphoid, triquetrum, and capitate to the lunate, stabilizing the reduction with pinning, and subsequent ligament and capsule repair are the necessary steps in treating these complex injuries. Associated styloid or carpal fractures are treated appropriately with either internal fixation or pinning, with bone grafting applied as necessary. In Stage III and IV injuries there is a consistent volar capsular rent that must be repaired. Additionally, the carpal tunnel should be released and the wrist immobilized after surgery. Despite early and anatomic reduction, most patients lose some degree of grip strength and motion, and also develop radiographic signs of arthritis and carpal collapse after these injuries; however, these clinical measurements and radiographic changes do not directly correlate with patient satisfaction or ability to return to work, especially when the carpal injury is an isolated problem [16].

Technique

Volarly, an extended carpal tunnel approach is used with care to identify and protect the palmar cutaneous nerve. The flexor tendons are retracted and the median nerve is inspected. With the nerve and flexor tendons retracted, the volar capsule is inspected. A transverse rent is consistently found within the volar capsule, extending from radial to ulnar. Most often this rent is proximal to the capitate, at the space of Poirier, between the RSC and LRL ligaments. If the lunate was not reduced, its distal articular surface can be visualized through this rent. The lunate is reduced by manually pushing it dorsally back between the capitate and radius. This is facilitated by manual longitudinal traction on the hand. The capsular rent is then repaired deep to its synovial covering with 3-0 nonabsorbable sutures (Fig. 9). It is important to note that the easily visualized portion of the rent is only its synovial covering, and that the important volar ligaments are deeper structures below this synovial layer and must be included as part of the repair. Special attention should be paid to the corners of the rent, to ensure

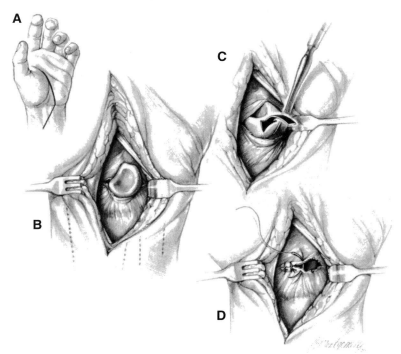

Fig. 9. Palmar approach—open reduction of dorsal perilunate-palmar lunate dislocation. (*A*) A proximally extended carpal tunnel incision is used. Care must be taken to avoid injury of the palmar cutaneous branch of the median nerve. (*B*) Once the flexor tendons are retracted radially, the palmar radiocarpal capsule is inspected. Usually a transverse rent coinciding with the space of Poirier, and across the palmar lunotriquetral ligaments, is found, whether the lunate is displaced into the carpal tunnel or not. (*C*) While an assistant applies longitudinal traction to the hand, the lunate is reduced. (*D*) The transverse derangement is repaired with nonabsorbable sutures. (*From* Garcia-Elias M. Carpal instability. In: Green DP, Hotchkiss RN, Pederson WC, et al, editors. Operative hand surgery. 5th edition. Philadelphia: Elsevier; 2005; with permission.)

that the ulnar LT and the radial RSC ligaments are included in the repair (Fig. 10).

After the volar rent has been repaired, a dorsal longitudinal incision is created over Lister's tubercle. The dissection continues between the third and fourth compartments. Silk sutures are placed in the retinacular flaps to aid in retraction. The fourth compartment is reflected ulnarly with its tendon sheath intact. The capsule is usually distended and filled with blood if it has not already been disrupted. Splitting the dorsal capsule in line with the fibers of the DRC, from the radius to the triquetrum and then to the capitate, allows for adequate visualization of the joint and a strong capsular repair during closure. The joint is thoroughly irrigated to remove any cartilaginous or osseous fragments. The full extent of injury is then assessed. Most often the SL ligament is avulsed from the lunate, and the LT ligament is avulsed from the triquetrum. The articular surfaces of the scaphoid, lunate, capitate, and radius are then inspected and documented, because full-thickness cartilage injuries are frequently found (Fig. 11).

A well-aligned lunate is the foundation upon which the carpus is then repaired. The lunate is reduced using a 0.062 Kirschner wire (K-wire) "joystick" placed halfway through the lunate from dorsal to volar. Once the lunate reduction has been confirmed under intraoperative fluoroscopy, it is stabilized with a temporary 0.062 K-wire from the radius to the lunate. The SL joint is then reduced by placing a joystick 0.062 K-wire in the scaphoid and correcting its orientation with the lunate. After the reduction is confirmed under fluoroscopy, the SL joint is stabilized using 0.045 K-wires; one or two wires from the scaphoid into the lunate, and another from the scaphoid into the capitate. These wires are safely placed using a 2 cm longitudinal incision over the anatomic snuffbox, just distal to the radial styloid to avoid injury to the radial artery and superficial radial nerve. A temporary joystick K-wire is then placed in the triquetrum to aid in reduction of the LT joint, and the joint is stabilized with a percutaneous 0.045 K-wire from the triquetrum to the lunate. Depending on surgeon preference, the lunocapitate (LC) joint can be further stabilized with two 0.045 K-wires from the capitate into the lunate. These wires can be placed retrograde through the capitate before reduction of the LC joint to facilitate their placement. Once the carpus is confirmed radiographically to be anatomically reduced and stabilized, the SL and LT ligaments are repaired using minisuture anchors (Fig. 12). At times the SL and LT ligaments are extensively damaged and primary repair is limited. In these cases, every attempt is made to repair the ligaments, and tacking them in place with suture anchors is acceptable and can still provide a good result. If there is not enough tissue remaining of the SL or LT ligaments, a primary stabilization procedure as described by Brunelli and Brunelli [17] or Linscheid and Dobyns [12] may be considered if repair is not possible.

Associated fractures of the carpal bones or radial styloid should be addressed before final joint reduction and fixation. Use of K-wires or screw fixation is equally acceptable and is based on surgeon preference. One should avoid excision of radial styloid fracture fragments because these fragments represent the attachment of the volar radiocarpal ligaments. Removal of these fragments may lead to radiocarpal instability postoperatively.

To ensure anatomic reduction, final radiographs should be obtained before closing the incisions. The wrist should be protected postoperatively in a short arm cast. Pins are usually removed at 8 to 10 weeks, followed by occupational therapy for range of motion and strengthening. A return to

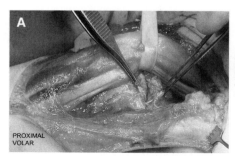
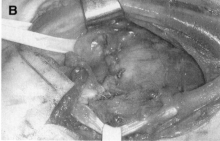

Fig. 10. (*A*) Volar capsular rent. (*B*) Capsular rent repaired with 3-0 nonabsorbable sutures. (Courtesy of Peter Carter, MD, Texas Scottish Rite Hospital, Dallas, TX.)

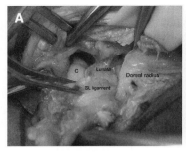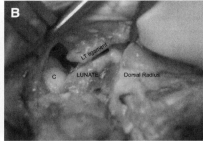

Fig. 11. Interosseous ligament avulsions. (*A*) Intraoperative inspection of the wrist usually reveals an avulsion of the SL ligament from the lunate. This is repaired with a minisuture anchor or bone tunnels. (*B*) Inspection of the LT ligament reveals avulsion of the LT ligament off the lunate, although it is more commonly found to have been avulsed from the triquetrum. C, capitate.

full activities of daily living is possible at 3 months, with sports and heavy labor restricted for at least 4 to 6 months. Because of the significant energy absorbed by the wrist in these injuries, some heavy laborers may have difficulty returning to full heavy activities until 1 year postoperatively.

Late presentation of perilunate dislocations

Occasionally patients may present well after the acute phase of their injury. The injury can be

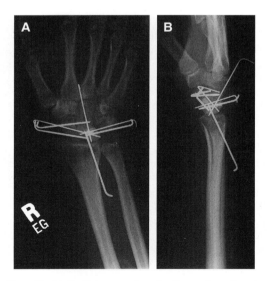

Fig. 12. (*A,B*) Intraoperative fixation of perilunate dislocation. AP and lateral radiographs of reduction and fixation of the carpal dislocation encountered in Fig. 6. Suture anchors were used to repair the SL and LT ligaments to the lunate. A K-wire from the radius to the lunate was used for temporary intraoperative fixation and was removed before closure.

missed acutely because of multiple other injuries or altered mental status. In this regard, chronic or late lunate dislocation is defined as greater than 6 weeks after injury [18]. Because of the length of time since injury, the surgeon is faced with the difficulty of addressing contracted soft tissues, cartilage loss, and possible carpal avascular necrosis. Although an attempt at closed reduction is warranted, it is most often unsuccessful and should only be attempted in the operating room with complete relaxation of the extremity and a clear operative plan if the location is unable to be reduced. A host of treatment options have been described, including open reduction and internal fixation, lunate excision, proximal row carpectomy, and wrist arthrodesis. Siegert and colleagues [10] reported on a series of 15 patients (10 dislocations, 5 fracture dislocations) who had delayed treatment. Six patients underwent open reduction internal fixation and all had satisfactory outcomes. Proximal row carpectomy and wrist arthrodesis were each performed in 2 patients, with all 4 patients obtaining acceptable results. Lunate excision alone was not found to be successful. The study authors found that open reduction, internal fixation (ORIF) is the procedure of choice unless faced with severe cartilage damage. If the repair fails, a salvage procedure can then be used.

Complications

Because of the amount of energy needed for carpal dislocations, significant injury to the bones, ligaments, and surrounding structures can result in complications despite optimal management. Stiffness, complex regional pain syndrome, lunate avascular changes, tendon rupture, and recurrence of instability have all been reported complications.

In one multicenter study [5], 56% of patients were found to have post-traumatic arthritis of the radiocarpal and midcarpal joints at an average of 6 years follow-up. Lunate changes with increased radiodensity may be noted during the first months after reduction; however, Kienböck's disease and lunate collapse are rare, with only a few cases reported in the literature [19].

Reverse perilunar dislocations

Much less common and less recognized are the ulnar sided perilunar injuries, which predominantly involve the LT, UT, and UL ligaments. Through biomechanical cadaver studies, a three-stage progressive perilunar instability pattern was noted to initiate on the ulnar side of the wrist [20]. Stage I involves a tear of the LT ligament. Stage II is disruption of the volar ulnar ligament complex and DRC and DIC ligaments. Stage III is a tear of the SL ligament and subsequent development of a perilunate dislocation. The mechanism for this injury pattern involves hyperextension, pronation, and ulnar deviation with an axial load, as in a fall on the outstretched hand. Treatment principles for these injuries are identical to perilunate dislocations and thus yield similar postoperative results.

Radiocarpal dislocations

Dissociation of the proximal row from the articular surface of the radius is an extremely rare injury, with an incidence of only 0.2% of all dislocations [21]. Usually associated with high-energy trauma, disruptions of the RSC, LRL, SRL, and DRC ligaments are required to produce a radiocarpal dislocation. Originally classified based on the presence of ligamentous instability within the proximal row, Type I injuries have an intact proximal row and Type II injuries have an associated tear of either the SL or LT ligament. The Type II injuries uniformly did poorly, according to Moneim and coworkers [21]. Dumontier and colleagues [22] proposed a new classification system based on the status of the radial styloid. In their classification, Group I dislocations had either no radial styloid fracture or only a small avulsion, whereas Group II dislocations had styloid fractures greater than one third the width of the scaphoid fossa. At follow-up, Dumontier and coworkers found that most patients in Group I had ulnar translation of the carpus, which they believed was due to avulsion and or attenuation

of the RSC and LRL ligaments from the radial styloid. The Group II patients maintained reduction after radial styloid fixation due to an intact RSC ligament [22].

Historically, a full array of treatment options has been attempted, from closed reduction and casting to arthrodesis. It is now generally recommended to perform an open reduction of these injuries with use of both volar and dorsal approaches, repair the volar radiocarpal ligaments and dorsal capsule, stabilize the joint with percutaneous pinning, and immobilize the wrist for up to 2 months [7]. Mudgal and colleagues [23] used this approach in 12 patients, and achieved satisfactory results in 8 of the 11 patients available for follow-up up at 36 months. Nyquist and Stern [24] reported on 10 open radiocarpal dislocations and noted that all had associated fractures and injuries to other organ systems. Seven of the 10 patients had median or ulnar nerve contusions, and all patients had evidence of some nerve dysfunction 15 months postinjury. Overall the prognosis for this injury is poor.

Axial dislocations

Axial-loading or longitudinal dislocations of the carpus describe carpal dislocations oriented along the long axis of the forearm. Also termed "capitohamate diastasis," "carpal arch disruption," or "columnar dislocations," they involve a traumatic disruption of the carpus in which it is longitudinally split and displaced. These are rare carpal dislocations, with an incidence of only 1.4% to 2.08% of patients with carpal fracture-dislocations or subluxations [7].

Mechanism of injury

Axial dislocations usually are the result of a high energy crush, twisting, or blast injury. Most often the result of industrial accidents secondary to various press and wringer machinery, the most common mechanism of injury is dorsopalmar compression of the wrist. Depending on the direction of force through the wrist, dislocations or sagittal fractures of the carpal bones will result [7]. Forces parallel to the intercarpal joints more often result in dislocation, whereas an increase in the obliquity of the applied force often leads to sagittal plane fractures (Fig. 13). Because of the significant crushing force necessary to produce these injuries, significant soft tissue injury almost always accompanies them.

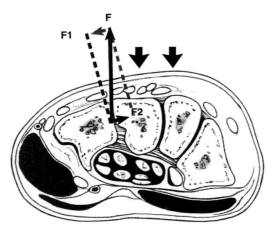

Fig. 13. Axial dislocation forces. When a dorsovolar compression force is applied to the distal carpal row, two vectors of force are created. A shear force tangential to the articular surface (*F1*) and a compressive force (*F2*) that is perpendicular to F1. If shear forces are higher at the joint, a dislocation occurs. If compressive forces are higher, a fracture results. Large arrows represent axial load. Dashed lines and smaller arrows are the vector forces. (*From* Tolo ET, Shin AY. Fracture dislocations of the carpus. In: Trumble TE, editor. Hand surgery update 3. Rosemont (IL): ASSH 2003; with permission)

Classification

After an extensive review of the 40 cases previously reported in the literature, and cases at their own institution, Garcia-Elias and coworkers [25] published a three-group classification of axial dislocations based on the direction of instability. In Group I, axial-ulnar dislocations, the carpus splits into two columns, in which the radial column is stable in relation to the radius, and the ulnar column, along with the metacarpals, displaces ulnarly and proximally; in Group II, axial-radial dislocations, the ulnar column is stable and the radial column and metacarpals displaces proximally and radially; and in Group III, combined axial-radial-ulnar dislocations, a mix of radial and ulnar column displacement is present (Fig. 14).

Treatment

The majority of axial-carpal dislocations are open dislocations with significant associated soft tissue injuries. Successful treatment of these complex injuries depends greatly on early and accurate assessment of the neurovascular and musculotendinous structures involved. Initial treatment should include a through debridement of severely contaminated and nonviable tissues. The need for

fasciotomies of the hand and forearm compartments should be carefully evaluated, both initially and throughout the perioperative period.

After thorough debridement, a dorsal longitudinal approach is used for carpal reduction, and reduction is maintained by percutaneous fixation with K-wires. Repair of intercarpal ligamentous injury is usually not possible because of the severity of soft tissue injury. If ligamentous repair is possible, use of suture anchors instead of drill holes reduces further trauma to the already injured tissues. An extended palmar approach should be used to evaluate the neurovascular and musculotendinous structures and for decompression of the carpal tunnel. All damaged structures should be repaired or grafted primarily, and covered with local or distant flaps if loose primary closure is not possible. Closed reduction and percutaneous pinning is possible; however, interposed soft tissue or fracture fragments may prevent anatomic reduction, necessitating open treatment.

Functional results and outcome after proper treatment of these injuries has been found to be more dependent on the associated soft tissue injuries than on the osseous injury. Studies have shown that lower energy injuries with less soft tissue damage have better functional results than higher energy injuries with greater soft tissue damage [25,26]. In a study by Garcia-Elias and colleagues [25], most of the patients had severe soft tissue injuries, with 4 of 13 patients having good results, 5 having fair results, and 4 having poor results. The researchers also noted that presence of a nerve injury and type of dislocation were most predictive of outcome.

Isolated carpal dislocations

Isolated dislocations of the carpal bones are relatively rare injuries. More often individual carpal bone dislocation is associated with a more global wrist dislocation pattern, such as progressive perilunate instability or the axial dislocations patterns. Because of their rarity, most of our information on isolated dislocations comes from a relatively small amount of case reports and technique papers. Although it is critically important to recognize the clinical and radiologic features of these injuries, definitive treatment recommendations have yet to be confirmed for many of these dislocations.

Lunate dislocation: palmar

The most common of the isolated carpal dislocations is the palmar lunate dislocation. As

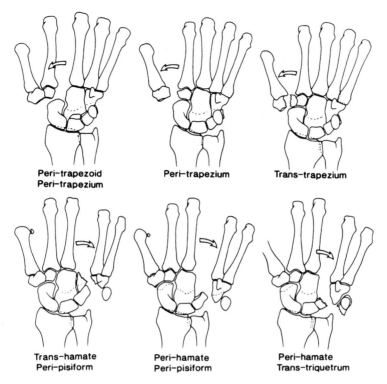

Peri-trapezoid
Peri-trapezium

Peri-trapezium

Trans-trapezium

Trans-hamate
Peri-pisiform

Peri-hamate
Peri-pisiform

Peri-hamate
Trans-triquetrum

Fig. 14. Axial carpal dislocation classification. (*Top*) Axial-radial dislocations: the radial part of the carpus is dislocated and unstable. (*Bottom*) Axial-ulnar dislocation: the ulnar part of the carpus is dislocated and unstable. Combined dislocation: in which both types of dislocation coexist in the same wrist. Arrows indicate the direction of the bony displacement as is evident with the bone separated from the rest of the hand. (*From* Garcia-Elias M, Geissler WB. Carpal instability. In: Green DP, Hotchkiss RN, Pederson WC, et al, editors. Operative hand surgery. 5th edition. Philadelphia: Elsevier; 2005; with permission.)

previously discussed in the section on perilunate dislocations, this injury is not an isolated dislocation, but represents Stage IV of the progressive perilunate instability pattern. This injury is addressed as outlined in the section on perilunate dislocations.

Lunate dislocation: dorsal

Although the majority of lunate dislocations are palmar, a significant palmar flexion force to the carpus or significant blow to the dorsum of the hand can result in palmar displacement of the carpus in relation to the lunate. This mechanism can result in a palmar perilunate or dorsal lunate dislocation [27]. Isolated dorsal lunate dislocation is extremely rare injury, with only four cases reported in the literature [28]. Swelling, tenderness, and a palpable firm mass on the dorsum of the wrist are found on clinical examination.

Standard radiographs reveal an overlap of the carpal bones on the PA view and a volarly tilted, dorsally displaced lunate on the lateral. For the four cases reported, two were seen acutely and two were seen late. Attempts at closed reduction failed in both acute injuries, and open reduction and fixation was required, with pinning of the lunate, capitate, scaphoid, and triquetrum. The two patients who presented late were treated with a proximal row carpectomy. One of the late presenting patients also underwent extensor tendon repair, because of multiple tendon ruptures caused by attrition of the tendons from the pressure of a dorsally dislocated lunate [28].

Scaphoid dislocation

Scaphoid dislocation is a rare injury, but has occurred with enough frequency to warrant its own classification: Type I, isolated anterolateral dislocation of the proximal pole; and Type II, scaphoid dislocation associated with an axial derangement of the capitate-hamate joint. Type I injuries are believed to result from violent forced hyperpronation to the extended and ulnarly deviated wrist while grasping a fixed object [29]. This force first causes an SL disruption followed by displacement of the scaphoid around the RC ligament. Another possibility is a self-reduced palmar perilunate dislocation, with the scaphoid remaining unreduced because of soft tissue interposition. Type II injuries fall under the realm of axial-ulnar dislocations (Fig. 15).

On examination of the wrist, swelling and a palpable firm mass either palmar, radial, or rarely dorsal to the radius are noted. Standard wrist series may reveal: (1) anterior, radial, or dorsal dislocation of the scaphoid; (2) normal axial alignment of the lunate on the PA view, but likely dorsal tilt of the lunate on the lateral view; and (3) proximal radial migration of the capitate.

Of the isolated cases reported, closed or open reduction and immobilization has been the mainstay of treatment, with most achieving good to excellent results [26,30]. Open reduction and ligament repair through a dorsal approach has more recently been advocated to facilitate and maintain anatomic reduction. In these instances, direct repair of the scapholunate interosseous ligament and scaphotrapezial ligament should be combined with K-wire fixation of the scaphotrapezial and scapholunate joints for duration of 8

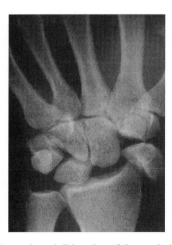

Fig. 15. Anterolateral dislocation of the scaphoid, Type I. (*From* Garcia-Elias M, Geissler WB. Carpal instability. In: Green DP, Hotchkiss RN, Pederson WC, et al, editors. Operative hand surgery. 5th edition. Philadelphia: Elsevier; 2005; with permission.)

to 10 weeks in a thumb spica cast. This approach has also achieved good to excellent results.

Closed reduction technique

As for most dislocations, an attempt at reduction requires a sufficient amount of muscle relaxation. Ten pounds of traction is applied with finger traps to further fatigue the forearm musculature. The thumb of the dominant hand is placed over the volar aspect of the radius and moved distally until resting on the proximal pole of the scaphoid. The finger traps are then removed and traction is maintained by the opposite hand. A dorsally directed pressure is applied to the proximal pole of the scaphoid as the wrist is ulnarly deviated. With this maneuver a reduction of the scaphoid is usually achieved.

Triquetrum

Only a few reported cases of isolated triquetrum dislocation have been detailed in the literature. With so few cases, definitive conclusions about the mechanism of injury and treatment outcomes are not available. Direct force to the triquetrum or wrist extension and ulnar deviation have been the proposed mechanisms of injury in a few of the reported cases [31,32]. Both volar and dorsal displacements have been seen, with volar displacement being associated with transient median nerve compression. In almost all cases the diagnosis was delayed, despite a tender palpable mass over the dislocation. Treatment has included fragment excision, ORIF, and reduction without fixation, all with reasonably good results [33,34].

Trapezoid

A very rare carpal dislocation, with fewer than 20 isolated dislocations without fracture reported in the literature. Because the trapezoid is wedge-shaped, wider dorsally, the trapezoid is most often displaced dorsal to the carpus, and is most often accompanied by the second metacarpal. Volar dislocation has been reported, and is believed to be the result of a direct force on the bone with midcarpal hyperextension. Closed reduction has been successfully accomplished with dorsal, but not volar, dislocations. Trapezoid excision has been associated with proximal migration of the second metacarpal, and AVN has been reported with open reduction and fixation. Good outcomes were achieved despite these radiographic complications.

Trapezium

Most dislocations of the trapezium are associated with first metacarpal dislocations, and are more accurately described as peritrapezial axial-radial dislocations [25]. True isolated dislocations of the trapezium are very rare, and are thought to be caused by a direct blow to the dorsolateral aspect of the wrist or a hyperextension-supination force to the wrist in radial deviation. In all instances the trapezium has displaced volarly and has been successfully treated with either open reduction or excision.

Hamate

Most reported cases of hamate dislocation are associated with fourth or fifth metacarpal displacement, and are appropriately classified as axial-ulnar dislocations [25]. True isolated hamate dislocations are very rare, with fewer than 20 cases in the literature [35]. Direct impact by a sharp tool penetrating the wrist and high energy traffic accidents have been the associated trauma. With both dorsal and volar dislocations reported, prompt treatment has achieved good results with both closed and open reduction with fixation, as well as fragment excision.

Pisiform dislocation

Isolated pisiform dislocation is an extremely rare injury, with only a handful of case reports in the literature [36]. The patient usually complains of ulnar palmar wrist pain with possible weakness of wrist flexion. A direct blow to the ulnar aspect of the hand or a strong traction on the flexor carpi ulnaris with the wrist in extension has been reported as possible mechanism of injury. Standard radiographs of PA, lateral, and 45° supinated views are usually clear in diagnosis. A carpal tunnel view is not required unless generalized pain and swelling raises suspicion of possible fracture of the hook of the hamate. Displacement of the pisiform has been reported distally, proximally, and ulnarly. With failure of both nonoperative and operative attempts at reduction, excision of the pisiform is recommended and is consistently the most successful treatment of pain [36].

Summary

Carpal dislocations are rare but significant injuries, and represent a variety of injury patterns. A through understanding of carpal anatomy, kinematics, and mechanisms of injury, and a high index of suspicion aid the surgeon in proper diagnosis and treatment of these significant injuries.

References

[1] Taleisnik J. The ligaments of the wrist. J Hand Surg [Am] 1976;1:110–8.

[2] Mayfield JK, Johnson RP, Kilcoyne RF. The ligaments of the human wrist and their functional significance. Anat Rec 1976;186:417–28.

[3] Berger RA. The ligaments of the wrist: a current overview of anatomy with considerations of their potential functions. Hand Clin 1997;13:63–82.

[4] Cooney WP, Bussey R, Dobyns JH, et al. Difficult wrist fractures: perilunate fracture-dislocations of the wrist. Clin Orthop 1987;214:136–47.

[5] Herzberg G, Comtet JJ, Linscheid RL, et al. Perilunate dislocations and fracture dislocations: a multicenter study. J Hand Surg [Am] 1993;18:768–79.

[6] Mayfield JK, Johnson RP, Kilcoyne RF. Carpal dislocations: pathomechanics and progressive perilunar instability. J Hand Surg [Am] 1980;5:226–41.

[7] Tolo ET, Shin AY. Fracture dislocations of the carpus. In: Trumble TE, editor. Hand surgery update 3. Rosemont (IL): ASSH; 2003. p. 192–3.

[8] Johnson RP. The acutely injured wrist and its residuals. Clin Orthop 1980;149:33–44.

[9] Witvoet J, Allieu Y. Lesions traumatiques fraiches [Acute traumatic injuries]. Rev Chir Orthop 1973; 59(Suppl 1):98–125 [in French].

[10] Siegert JJ, Frassica FJ, Amadio PC. Treatment of chronic perilunate dislocations. J Hand Surg [Am] 1988;13:206–12.

[11] Dobyns JH, Swanson GE. A 19 year-old with multiple fractures. Minn Med 1973;56:143–9.

[12] Linscheid RL, Dobyns JH. Treatment of scapholunate dissociation. Hand Clin 1992;8:645–52.

[13] Sotereanos DG, Mitsionis GJ, Giannakopoulos PN, et al. Perilunate dislocation and fracture-dislocation: a critical analysis of the volar-dorsal approach. J Hand Surg [Am] 1997;22:49–56.

[14] Green DP, O'Brien ET. Open reduction of carpal dislocations: indications and operative techniques. J Hand Surg [Am] 1978;3:250–65.

[15] Minami A, Kaneda K. Repair and/or reconstruction of scapholunate interosseous ligament in lunate and perilunate dislocations. J Hand Surg [Am] 1993; 18(6):1099–106.

[16] Hildebrand KA, Ross DC, Patterson SD, et al. Dorsal perilunate dislocations and fracture-dislocations: questionnaire, clinical, and radiographic evaluation. J Hand Surg [Am] 2000;25(6):1069–79.

[17] Brunelli GA, Brunelli GR. A new surgical technique for carpal instability with scapho-lunar dislocation: eleven cases. Ann Chir Main Memb Super 1995;14: 207–13.

[18] Mueller JJ. Avascular necrosis and collapse of the lunate following a volar perilunate dislocation. A case report and review of this complication in

dislocations of the wrist. Orthopedics 1984;7:
1009–14.

[19] Shin AY, Battaglia MJ, Bishop AT. Lunotriquetral
instability: diagnosis and treatment. J Am Acad
Orthop Surg 2000;8(3):170–9.

[20] Dunn WA. Fractures and dislocations of the carpus.
Surg Clin North Am 1972;52(6):1513–38.

[21] Moneim MS, Bolger JT, Omber GE. Radiocarpal
dislocation-classification and rationale for management. Clin Orthop 1985;192:199–209.

[22] Dumontier C, Meyer zu Reckendorf G, Sautet A,
et al. Radiocarpal dislocations: classification and
proposal for treatment. A review of twenty-seven
cases. J Bone Joint Surg Am 2001;83(2):212–8.

[23] Mudgal CS, Psenica J, Jupiter JB. Radiocarpal
fracture-dislocation. J Hand Surg [Br] 1999;24(1):
92–8.

[24] Nyquist SR, Stern PJ. Open radiocarpal fracture-
dislocations. J Hand Surg [Am] 1984;9(5):707–10.

[25] Garcia-Elias M, Dobyns JH, Cooney WP III, et al.
Traumatic axial dislocations of the carpus. J Hand
Surg [Am] 1989;14(3):446–57.

[26] Garcia-Elias M, Bishop AT, Dobyns JH, et al.
Transcarpal carpometacarpal dislocations, excluding the thumb. J Hand Surg [Am] 1990;15(4):
531–41.

[27] Minami A, Ogino T, Mamada M. Rupture of extensor tendons associated with a palmar perilunar dislocation. J Hand Surg [Am] 1989;14:843–7.

[28] Schwartz MG, Green SM, Coville FA. Dorsal dislocations of the lunate with multiple extensor tendon
ruptures. J Hand Surg [Am] 1990;15:132–3.

[29] Maki NJ, Chuinard RG, D'Ambrosia R. Isolated,
complete radial dislocation of the scaphoid. A case
report and review of the literature. J Bone Joint
Surg Am 1982;64:615–6.

[30] Cherif MR, Ben Ghozlen R, Chehimi A, et al. Isolated dislocation of the carpal scaphoid. A case report with review of the literature. Chir Main 2002;
21(5):305–8 [in French].

[31] Frykman E. Dislocation of the triquetrum. Case Report. Scand J Plast Reconstr Surg 1980;14:205–7.

[32] Soucacos PN, Hartofilakidis-Garofalidis GC. Dislocation of the triangular bone. Report of a case.
J Bone Joint Surg Am 1981;63:1012–4.

[33] Bieber EJ, Weiland AJ. Traumatic dorsal dislocation of the triquetrum: a case report. J Hand Surg
[Am] 1984;9:840–2.

[34] Goldberg B, Heller AP. Dorsal dislocation of the triquetrum with rotary subluxation of the scaphoid.
J Hand Surg [Am] 1987;12:119–22.

[35] Aieren J, Agnes A, Muller JM. Isolated dislocation
of the hamate bone. Case report and review of the literature. Arch Orthop Trauma Surg 2000;120(9):
535–7.

[36] Levante S, Ebelin M. Traumatic dislocation of the
pisiform bone: a case report and review of the literature. Chir Main 2002;21(4):264–8 [in French].

ELSEVIER
SAUNDERS

Hand Clin 22 (2006) 501–516

HAND
CLINICS

Carpal Fractures Excluding the Scaphoid

Mordechai Vigler, MD[a], Alberto Aviles, MD[b], Steve K. Lee, MD[a],*

[a]*Hand Surgery Service, New York University Hospital for Joint Diseases Orthopaedic Institute,
Department of Orthopaedic Surgery, The New York University School of Medicine, 301 East 17th Street,
New York, NY 10003, USA*
[b]*Hand Surgery Service, The Institute of Plastic and Reconstructive Surgery,
The New York University School of Medicine, 550 1st Avenue, New York, NY 10016, USA*

According to ICD-9-CM diagnostic codes in 1998, an estimated 188,000 to 226,000 carpal fractures were treated in emergency rooms across the United States [1]. Although the scaphoid accounts for 62% to 87% of carpal fractures, clinicians should not underestimate the frequency by which the remainder of the carpus is fractured. These injuries are often difficult to diagnose and the treatments rendered inadequate and delayed.

In recent literature, the incidence of carpal fractures in overall hand injuries has ranged from 8% to 19% since 1990 [2–4]. The frequency of such fractures has not changed significantly since Emmet and Breck [5] reported a 17% incidence in 1958. Nonscaphoid fractures account for 3.2% to 7.7% of these injuries. A breakdown between the proximal and distal row separately demonstrates that fractures of the distal row account for 0.8% to 1.4% of all hand injuries. The hamate is injured most frequently in the distal row, whereas the triquetrum is the second most commonly injured behind the scaphoid with respect to the proximal row [2,3]. Triquetral fractures vary from 4% to 20% with different studies, whereas the remaining carpal bones (trapezium, hamate, capitate, lunate, pisiform, and trapezoid) are less frequently injured, with a range of 0.2% to 3% [2,3,6–9]. The rarity of such fractures offers few outcomes data.

The strategy behind carpal fracture treatment is to make accurate diagnoses, determine the degree of displacement, severity of symptoms, and to address concomitant injuries. Treatment should be directed not only at the fracture, but possible surrounding associated injuries. Carpal fractures are relatively uncommon, but care must be given to diagnose and treat these injuries appropriately. Misdiagnosed and untreated carpal fractures may lead to nonunion, malunion, avascular necrosis, carpal instability, articular incongruity with resultant osteoarthrosis, neurovascular compression, or late tendon rupture, among other conditions [7–9].

Fractures of the capitate

Fractures of the capitate are rare and account for only 1.3% of all carpal fractures [10]. Most of these fractures occur in association with additional carpal pathology, particularly scaphoid fractures; isolated fractures of the capitate comprise only 0.3% of carpal injuries [10].

Harrigan [11] reported on the first case of an isolated capitate fracture in 1908. In 1962, Adler and Shaftan [12] reported on 48 cases of isolated capitate fractures. Of the 16 cases with known treatment, 14 were treated by immobilization and 2 by excision. Results were reported in only 8 cases; five patients had a "good" result and three had a "poor" result. One of these three underwent capitolunate fusion. Unfortunately, many of these cases had incomplete data, and no data were available regarding the incidence of nonunion.

Since 1962, only 25 cases of isolated capitate fractures have been reported [10,13–27]. These reports emphasize that early diagnosis is important because delayed treatment may lead to avascular necrosis (AVN), nonunion, and post-traumatic arthritis [13].

* Corresponding author.
E-mail address: steve.lee@nyumc.org (S.K. Lee).

The low incidence of isolated capitate fractures is postulated to be because of its anatomical position; the capitate is protected from injury by its surrounding bones, namely the third and fourth metacarpal, hamate, lunate, scaphoid, and trapezoid bones. In addition, these fractures may be underdiagnosed; little, if any, displacement of fracture fragments occur, because of stabilization by intracarpal ligaments [13,28]. The fracture may also be initially missed because of a paucity of symptoms and a radiographically occult fracture.

Studies by Gelberman and colleagues [29–31] demonstrated that the capitate is vulnerable to post-traumatic avascular necrosis because of its blood supply. The capitate has a dorsal blood supply with two to four vessels entering the distal two thirds on its concave surface. These vessels supply the body and head in 67% of specimens. One to three vessels enter from the palmar side. The blood vessels to the head of the capitate originate entirely from the palmar surface in 33% of specimens. This retrograde blood flow (similar to the scaphoid) is believed to place the capitate with a waist fracture at risk for AVN [29–31].

Of the three mechanisms considered to cause isolated fractures of the capitate, the more frequent is a fall on the palm with the wrist extended [12,32]. Biomechanical cadaver studies have demonstrated that the dorsal lip of the radius may strike the capitate with hyperextension [22]. The other causes are axial load or a direct blow over the dorsum of the wrist.

Early diagnosis cannot be overemphasized. Unfortunately, the frequent paucity of symptoms contributes to the possible delay in diagnosis [28,33,34]. If an isolated nondisplaced capitate fracture is missed and not immobilized, the proximal segment may rotate with wrist movements producing AVN or nonunion caused by interruption of the vascularization of the head (proximal pole) [35].

When a displaced capitate fracture occurs as an isolated injury, plain radiographs are usually diagnostic (Fig. 1A,B); however, nondisplaced isolated capitate fractures may be radiographically occult [13,36,37]. Multiple radiographic studies may be required for diagnosis. PA radial and ulnar deviation views may help make nondisplaced capitate waist fractures visible on plain radiographs. Hopkins and Ammann [15] found that early diagnosis of a capitate fracture could be obtained with a 99M–Tc-methylene disphosphonate nuclear medicine bone scan and confirmed with CT or MRI. Other authors [13,37–40] have also reported the usefulness of CT and MRI [31].

Calandruccio and Duncan [13] reported a case of isolated capitate fracture in which initial plain radiographs were considered normal. Treatment was delayed until the fracture was diagnosed with the use of MRI. The authors prefer using MRI to confirm an occult capitate fracture.

Nondisplaced isolated capitate fractures should be treated with short-arm thumb spica cast immobilization for 6 to 8 weeks [33]. Displaced fractures require anatomic reduction to restore normal carpal kinematics [16]. In a longterm follow-up study of capitate fractures, Rand and coworkers [10] recommended anatomic reduction (by open technique if necessary) and immobilization until the fracture united. Volk and colleagues [41] reported an excellent outcome with open reduction and stabilization using a Herbert screw or Kirshner wires (K-wires). Internal fixation by K-wires or Herbert screws has also been reported by others [16].

The most substantial and under recognized complication of isolated capitate fractures is that of nonunion. Of the 25 cases of isolated capitate fractures reported in the literature since 1962, 14 (56%) developed nonunion [10,18,19,22,23,33,42]. Yoshihara and coworkers [22] reported 12 cases of nonunion in the literature, and reported the incidence of nonunion amongst isolated capitate fractures as being 19.6%. This percentage took into account the 48 cases reported by Adler and Shaftan in 1962 [12] and assumed that none of them developed nonunion, although this was not specifically stated.

Of the 14 cases of nonunion in the literature, the average patient age was 27 years old, ranging from 13 to 54 years. All were diagnosed late, with the average period from injury to definitive diagnosis being 1 year and 11 months (range 3 months to 7 years). The regions of nonunion were the proximal third in 3 cases, the middle third in 10 cases, and the distal third in one case. Of the 14 cases of nonunion, 8 did not receive initial treatment after injury because of missed diagnoses. The other 5 were initially treated with immobilization because of suspected contusion or "sprain," but the fractures failed to unite. The details of the remaining 1 case as to initial treatment are unknown. The treatment in 10 cases was cancellous or corticocancellous bone grafting, with or without screw fixation, and observation in 4 cases [27]. Nine out of 10 operated cases obtained union. The other cases did not achieve union. Rico and colleagues [28] reported that cancellous or corticocancellous bone grafting after correction of the rotation of the fragments

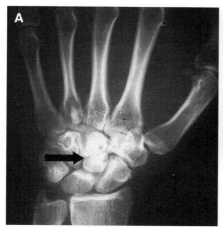
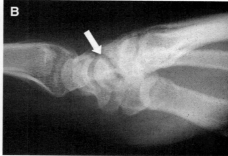

Fig. 1. (*A*) Capitate waist fracture (*arrow*), posteroanterior (PA) radiograph. (*B*) Capitate waist fracture (*arrow*), lateral radiograph. (Courtesy of Martin A. Posner, MD, New York, NY.)

achieved bone union and restored the length of the capitate, but with some reduction in mobility.

The long-term probability of arthritis after an isolated capitate nonunion is unknown and has not been reported; however, 66% of patients who had scaphocapitate syndrome developed post-traumatic arthritis [10].

AVN of the capitate after an isolated capitate fracture is rare, with only three cases reported in the literature [15,24,43]. Grend and coworkers [35] reported that a fracture through the capitate jeopardizes the blood supply to the proximal portion of the bone by interference with the intraosseous circulation, thus potentially resulting in AVN.

The high incidence of nonunion of isolated capitate fractures (56%) has not been previously recognized. All cases were associated with late diagnosis, highlighting the importance of early diagnosis and treatment. A patient suspected of having a capitate fracture based on clinical examination and history should undergo further imaging with MRI when initial radiographs are negative. Nondisplaced fractures warrant 6 to 8 weeks in a short-arm thumb spica cast. Displaced fractures require closed versus open reduction and internal fixation (ORIF), with K-wires or headless compression screws, depending on the individual fracture pattern. Box 1 provides diagnosis and treatment guidelines.

Fractures of the pisiform

Fracture of the pisiform is uncommon, the estimated incidence being less than 1% of all carpal bone fractures [44]. A literature review in all languages reveals 137 reported cases of pisiform fracture. The pisiform bone is a sesamoid bone and is the only carpal bone into which a tendon, the flexor carpi ulnaris (FCU), inserts; it articulates with the triquetrum dorsally and serves as the attachment of the transverse carpal

---

Box 1. Capitate summary

Classification [95]
Type 1. Transverse body
Type 2. Transverse proximal pole (waist) (Fig. 1)
Type 3. Coronal oblique
Type 4. Parasagittal

Mechanisms
1. Hyperextension with capitate striking distal radius
2. Axial load
3. Direct blow

Treatment
- Nondisplaced: Short arm thumb spica cast × 6–8 weeks
- Displaced: CRIF vs ORIF (K-wires, headless compression screws)

Abbreviations: CRIF, closed reduction internal fixation; K-wire, Kirschner wire; ORIF, open reduction internal fixation.

ligament and the FCU tendon, and the origin of the abductor digiti minimi muscle [45]. The FCU tendon continues distally as the pisohamate and pisometacarpal ligaments. The pisiform is the last carpal bone to ossify between the ages of 8 and 12 years. There may be multiple centers of ossification, giving it a fragmented appearance before age 12 years [44]. This normal variant must be distinguished from a fracture [46].

The mechanism of injury is most commonly direct trauma to the hypothenar eminence or avulsion when the FCU resists forcible hyperextension of the wrist, resulting in an osteochondral or avulsion fracture [44,47,48]. This can also be achieved by straining to lift a heavy object. A third mechanism postulated is repetitive trauma causing vascular disruption, microfractures, and then a complete fracture line [49].

The diagnosis is often missed because the adjacent bones obscure clear radiographic imaging of the pisiform on standard views [44,49–52]. Lacey and Hodge [53] highlighted the importance of obtaining a reverse oblique wrist radiograph with the wrist in supination. The pisiform fracture was only seen on this view in the two cases they presented. Fleege and coworkers [44] reported on 10 pisiform fractures, only 5 of which could be diagnosed on PA radiographs. Sagittal and transverse pisiform fractures may be seen on the PA view. The carpal tunnel view may also be a useful adjuvant view to diagnose pisiform fractures (Fig. 2). It profiles the pisiform with or without the pisotriquetral joint [43]. Abbit and Riddervold [54] presented a case of pisiform fracture that was not recognized on standard wrist views, but was diagnosed on the carpal tunnel view. It must be borne in mind that the carpal tunnel view may be unattainable in the acute setting because dorsiflexion is limited by pain. Because of difficulty with diagnosis, the true incidence of pisiform

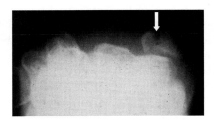

Fig. 2. Pisiform sagittal fracture (*arrow*), carpal tunnel view radiograph. (Courtesy of Martin A. Posner, MD, New York, NY.)

fractures is probably higher than that reported in the literature.

When plain radiographs remain nondiagnostic in a patient clinically suspected of a pisiform fracture, CT scan of the wrist is the study of choice. The importance of early diagnosis was emphasized by Fleege and coworkers [44]. Missed or delayed treatment of pisiform fractures may result in malunion or nonunion. This may manifest as chronic pain, grip weakness, or limitation of movement [45]. Later sequelae are pisotriquetral chondromalacia, subluxation, and osteoarthritis if the articular surface is poorly aligned [47,55].

Associated ulnar nerve palsy

The pisiform forms the ulnar wall of the Guyon tunnel, which contains the ulnar nerve and artery. It is because of this proximity that ulnar nerve palsy can be associated with pisiform fracture. Matsunaga and colleagues [56] described two patients who had pisiform fracture resulting in ulnar nerve palsy. Both patients had multiple injuries resulting in delayed diagnosis of the fracture and subsequent ulnar nerve palsy. Tenderness over the pisiform and normal dorsal sensibility of the ring and small fingers were diagnostic for an ulnar nerve injury at Guyon's canal. Both patients underwent excision of the entire pisiform; one had full recovery of ulnar nerve function and one had partial recovery. Two other cases of associated ulnar nerve palsy reported by Howard in 1961 [57] and Israeli and coworkers in 1982 [49] spontaneously resolved; one following nonoperative treatment with cast immobilization and the other having no treatment.

Because of the rarity of acutely diagnosed pisiform fracture, there are no well-defined guidelines for optimal treatment. Most acute pisiform fractures are treated by immobilization with a cast [5]. Israeli and colleagues [49] recommended immobilization for 6 weeks. Lacey and Hodge [53] suggest immobilization in a spica cast for 1 month and excision for those patients failing this period of immobilization. Georgoulis and colleagues [58] reported on four cases of pisiform fracture and recommended that acute fractures be treated with immobilization for 4 weeks. They emphasized that excision of the pisiform is not indicated in an acute injury.

For comminuted pisiform fractures, some authors feel that successful union is essentially precluded, and that early excision facilitates an uncomplicated recovery [59]. Geissler [60] recommended early excision for comminuted pisiform fractures in athletes to promote an uncomplicated recovery and early return to sport. The authors' preferred method of treatment is immobilization in a short-arm cast for 4 to 6 weeks for acute non- to minimally displaced fractures. Treatment for widely displaced fractures greater than 2–3 mm with loss of flexor carpi ulnaris (FCU) continuity should be pisiform excision and FCU repair. Pisiform excision is the treatment for cases of chronic, symptomatic nonunion, or pisotriquetral arthritis. Carroll and Coyle [48] reported complete relief in 65 out of 67 patients treated by excision of pisiform for pisotriquetral joint arthritis. Although this series did not include pisiform fractures, it nonetheless is suggestive of the efficacy of pisiform excision for chronic cases. No significant adverse effect on wrist function has been shown by total pisiform excision [45,53,55,61].

The indication for ulnar nerve exploration at Guyon's canal in patients who have pisiform fracture has not been clearly defined. According to Israeli and coworkers [49], the damage to the ulnar nerve is usually neurapraxia, and nerve palsy should improve within 6 weeks. Nerve exploration is indicated when nerve function does not improve or it deteriorates. Matsunaga and colleagues [56] recommended nerve exploration if sensory deficits persist for several months or if the ulnar nerve palsy is progressive. They suggested that resolution of the palsy without surgery is unlikely to occur inside Guyon's canal in the presence of a compressive lesion such as that caused by fractured fragments. The authors' approach is to observe if the fracture is nondisplaced. If there is no resolution after 8 to 12 weeks, we decompress Guyon's canal and perform a total pisiform excision. If symptoms worsen at any point, or if there are fracture fragments in Guyon's canal with ulnar nerve palsy, we prefer early exploration, decompression, and total pisiform excision.

Technique of pisiform excision

A palmar approach is used with a curvilinear or zigzag incision slightly radial to the palpable pisiform. The ulnar nerve is exposed and the pisohamate ligament divided to decompress Guyon's canal. This maneuver reduces the development of secondary compression in Guyon's canal postoperatively. If the fracture is old and the FCU tendon is intact, a longitudinal incision is made in the tendon and periosteum and the pisiform is shelled out. The tendon and skin are then closed and a soft dressing applied. If the injury has resulted in a transverse fracture with a wide

diastasis, the FCU will not be intact; in such cases the transverse rent in the tendon is used to visualize and shell out the two halves of the pisiform. The tendon is then repaired [62]. Box 2 provides diagnosis and treatment guidelines.

Fractures of the trapezium

Fractures of the trapezium account for 3% to 5% of all carpal fractures [63,64]. These fractures are significant injuries when displaced because they affect the important trapeziometacarpal joint of the thumb. Inadequate treatment can lead to permanent impairment based on the substantial forces experienced at the trapeziometacarpal joint in pinch and grip [65].

Isolated fractures of the trapezium are uncommon [66]. McGuigan and Culp [67] reported on three isolated fractures in a multicenter retrospective study of 11 patients who had intra-articular fractures of the trapezium. Two of these

---

Box 2. Pisiform summary

Classification [95]
Type 1. Transverse (most common)
Type 2. Sagittal (Fig. 2)
Type 3. Comminuted
Type 4. Pisotriquetral impaction

Mechanisms
1. Direct blow
2. Eccentric FCU load
3. Repetitve trauma

Special radiographs (CT scan still often necessary)
1. Reverse oblique (45° supination)
2. Carpal tunnel view

Treatment
1. Acute:
   - Non- to minimally displaced: SAC × 4–6 weeks
   - Widely displaced with loss of FCU continuity: pisiform excision and FCU repair
2. Chronic, symptomatic nonunion or arthritic pisotriquetral joint: pisiform excision

---

Abbreviations: FCU, flexor carpi ulnaris; SAC, short-arm cast.

were caused by motor vehicle collisions and one was caused by a fall. Four out of 11 patients had associated Bennett fractures and 2 had associated radius fractures. One patient had a hamate fracture and the remaining 2 patients presented with associated clavicle and scapula fractures respectively. The association between trapezial and Bennett fractures was first noted by Cordery and Ferrer-Torrells [68], who wrote "fracture of the first metacarpal is the most common associated injury."

Trapezial fractures fall into two main categories: fractures involving the palmar ridge (Fig. 3) and fractures through the body. The mechanism of injury for palmar ridge fractures is usually a fall on the outstretched palm, with fracture either by direct blow or indirect avulsion. The avulsion injury is caused by a sudden tension force applied to the transverse carpal ligament as the thenar and hypothenar eminences diverge. Trapezial palmar ridge fractures are subdivided into type I fractures, located at the base of the ridge, and type II fractures, located at the tip of the ridge (Fig. 4) [69]. Both types of fractures are associated with local tenderness. Pain with resisted wrist flexion is common because of the close proximity of the flexor carpi radialis tendon to the fracture site.

Trapezial body fractures may be are divided into vertical (Fig. 5), horizontal, dorsoradial tuberosity, and comminuted. The mechanism of injury is either axial load through the thumb metacarpal or hyperextension-abduction of the thumb that forces the wrist into a position of maximum radial deviation. The trapezium is wedged between the first metacarpal and styloid process of the radius; the styloid, functioning as an anvil, fractures the trapezium [70,71]. The fracture is

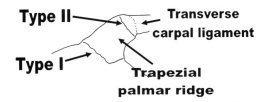

Fig. 4. Trapezial palmar ridge fractures, types I and II (*arrows*). (*Adapted from* Palmer AK. Trapezial ridge fractures. J Hand Surg [Am] 1981;6:564.)

generally located in the middle of the bone. The lateral fragment remains tethered to the first metacarpal and is often displaced radially and proximally by the pull of the abductor pollicis longus, similar to the mechanism that contributes to a displaced Bennett fracture. Horizontal fractures through the trapezium are rare [72].

Trapezial fractures, regardless of location, are frequently overlooked because of inadequate radiographs [66,73]. PA and lateral views fail to show the entire body of the bone: the PA view because of superimposition by the trapezoid and base of the second metacarpal, and the lateral view because of superimposition by the hook of the hamate. To visualize the entire body of the trapezium, an oblique radiographic view is necessary. One such view is the Bett's view, also known as the Gedda view in Europe, which is obtained by lifting the elbow off the table, hypothenar eminence off the cassette (on a wedge) with the thumb abducted and extended, hand semipronated from lateral, and directing the radiographic beam at the scaphoid-trapezium-trapezoid joints. In this view, all four articulations of the trapezium are visualized without overlap from the surrounding bones [74]. Visualization of the palmar ridge requires a carpal tunnel view. If a fracture is suspected but not adequately visualized by plain

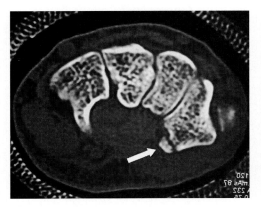

Fig. 3. Trapezial palmar ridge fracture (*arrow*), type I at the base, axial CT.

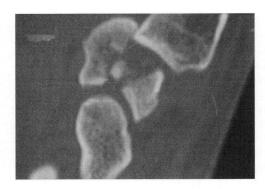

Fig. 5. Trapezium vertical body fracture.

radiographs, a CT scan may confirm the diagnosis and aid in treatment planning (see Fig. 3) [66,75].

Treatment of nondisplaced palmar ridge fractures is short-arm thumb spica cast immobilization for 4 to 6 weeks. Type I fractures through the base of the ridge heal more predictably than type II fractures at the tip of the ridge. For symptomatic nonunion of palmar ridge fractures, excision of the bony fragment is indicated [69].

Treatment of nondisplaced body fractures is short-arm thumb spica cast immobilization for 4 to 6 weeks. For displaced fractures, Cordrey and Ferrer-Torells [68] recommend ORIF of trapezial fractures to restore articular anatomy. Foster and Hastings [76] recommend closed reduction and pinning or ORIF to restore articular congruity. Walker and colleagues [77] advocate ORIF for all displaced fractures. Similarly, Pointu and co-workers [78] recommend reduction and fixation for "unstable fractures".

For comminuted fractures of the trapezium, Jones and Ghorbal [71] showed dismal results in three patients treated with casting. Gelberman and colleagues [79] demonstrated successful treatment with a system of oblique traction. Recommended indication for surgery by McGuigan and Culp [67] is either an articular step-off less than 2 mm or carpometacarpal subluxation. They reported on three patients who had isolated comminuted trapezial fractures and who had good results at average follow-up of 47 months, following ORIF. Two patients had K-wire insertion and one was fixed with a Herbert screw. The authors prefer distraction using a transmetacarpal 0.062 inch K-wire from the first to second metacarpal shafts, or external fixation to unload the joint in conjunction with ORIF. Box 3 provides diagnosis and treatment guidelines.

Fractures of the lunate

Isolated acute fractures secondary to trauma are rare, and if one is suspected, a diagnosis of Kienböck's disease should be entertained. Anatomically, 70% of the lunate sits on the radius, whereas 30% articulates with the triangular fibrocartilage complex (TFCC). During extreme dorsiflexion and ulnar deviation, in which the radius and capitate impart a large force onto the lunate, a fracture may result [7,9]. In 50% of lunate fractures, associated injuries to the distal radius, carpus, or metacarpals can occur. Appropriate studies are necessary to visualize such fractures. Oblique films may reveal avulsion fractures;

Box 3. Trapezium summary

Classification [95]
Type 1. Vertical intra-articular (Fig. 5)
Type 2. Horizontal (rare)
Type 3. Dorsoradial tuberosity
Type 4. Palmar ridge (Fig. 4)
  a. Type I. Base (Fig. 3)
  b. Type II. Tip
Type 5. Comminuted

Mechanisms
Type 1. Axial compression from 1st metacarpal
Type 2. Horizontal shear
Type 3. Vertical shear on radial styloid
Type 4. Direct blow or avulsion of transverse carpal ligament
Type 5. Axial compression from 1st metacarpal

Special radiographs (CT scan still often necessary)
1. Bett's (or Gedda's) view (see text)
2. Carpal tunnel view (for palmar ridge fractures)

Treatment
Body:
- Nondisplaced: SATSC × 4–6 weeks
- Displaced: CRIF vs ORIF (Wagner approach)
- Comminuted: ORIF combined with traction pin (1st to 2nd metacarpal) or external fixator

Palmar ridge:
Type I. SATSC × 4–6 weeks (usually heal)
Type II. SATSC × 4–6 weeks (often do not heal; excise if symptomatic)

Abbreviation: SATSC, short-arm thumb spica cast.

---

however, a CT scan is often needed to define subtle injuries [6,7,9,80].

Gelberman and coworkers [81] studied the vascular anatomy of the lunate and concluded that the proximal radial aspect of the bone is the least perfused. It is this segment in which a fracture may disrupt what little blood supply is present. Teisen and Hjarbaek [6] classified lunate fractures

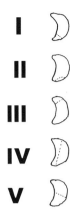

Fig. 6. Teisen and Hjarbaek classification of lunate fractures, Types I–V. I. Volar pole (most common), II. Chip, III. Dorsal pole, IV. Sagittal body, V. Transverse body. (*Adapted from* Teisen H, Hjarbaek J. Classification of fresh fractures of the lunate. J Hand Surg [Br] 1988;13:459.)

as follows: I. Volar pole (most common), II. Chip, III. Dorsal pole, IV. Sagittal body, and V. Transverse body (Fig. 6). Type I or volar pole fractures are considered the most common, whereas those through the body are the least frequent [6,9].

For nondisplaced fractures or small avulsions, treatment is immobilization in a short-arm cast for 6 weeks. Displaced fractures and fractures associated with multiple injuries usually require ORIF [6,7,9,80]. If the patient presents with a chronic lunate injury or severe comminution, a salvage procedure may be necessary to relieve symptoms, including partial fusion or proximal row carpectomy (Figs. 7A–F). Box 4 provides diagnosis and treatment guidelines.

Fractures of the triquetrum

Triquetral fractures occur in three patterns: dorsal cortical fractures (Fig. 8), body fractures,

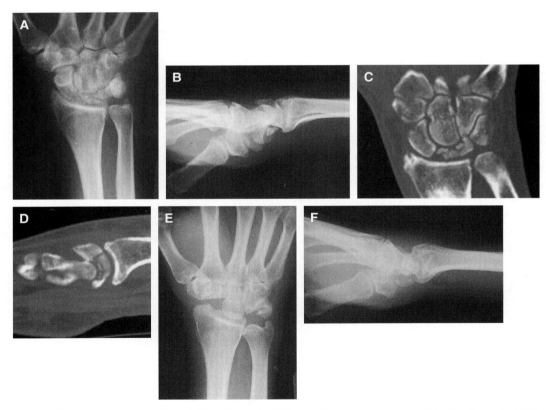

Fig. 7. (*A*) Lunate fracture, comminuted, PA radiograph. (*B*) Lunate fracture, comminuted, lateral radiograph. (*C*) Lunate fracture, comminuted, coronal CT. (*D*) Lunate fracture, comminuted, sagittal CT. (*E*) Proximal row carpectomy, PA radiograph. (*F*) Proximal row carpectomy, lateral radiograph.

Box 4. Lunate summary

Classification [6] (Fig. 6)
Type I. Palmar pole (most common)
Type II. Osteochondral chip
Type III. Dorsal pole
Type IV. Sagittal-oblique body
Type V. Transverse body [6]
Type VI. Comminuted (Fig. 7)

Mechanisms
Type I. Hyperextension, possible ligamentous avulsion fracture
Type II. Shear
Type III. Shear from capitate or ligamentous (scapholunate) avulsion fracture
Type IV. Shear during radiocarpal fracture-dislocation
Type V.
  a. Hyperextension with capitate forcing dorsal half of lunate into extension and short
     radiolunate ligament forcing palmar half into flexion. Fracture in mid-section results
  b. Shear with palmar displacement of capitate in palmar perilunate injury
Type VI. Axial compression between radius and capitate

Treatment
Type I.
  - Nondisplaced and small, no instability: SAC × 6 weeks
  - Large and/or displaced, or signs of carpal instability (usually VISI as lunate is unlinked
    from triquetrum): ORIF
Type II. SAC × 4–6 weeks, arthroscopic debridement or excision if remains symptomatic
Type III.
  - Nondisplaced and small, no instability: SAC × 6 weeks
  - Large and/or displaced, or signs of carpal instability (usually DISI as lunate is unlinked
    from scaphoid): ORIF
Type IV. ORIF if displaced
Type V. ORIF if displaced or carpal instability
Type VI. Severe comminution or chronic (without capitate / lunate fossa arthrosis): Proximal
  row carpectomy

Abbreviations: DISI, dorsal intercalated segmental instability; VISI, volar intercalated segmental instability.

---

and palmar cortical fractures. De Beer and Hudson [82] reported that the dorsal avulsion fracture accounted for 93% of all triquetral fractures. Clinically, there is localized edema over the ulnar aspect of the wrist as well as point tenderness over the triquetrum. For dorsal cortical fractures, pain is accentuated with palmar flexion as the dorsal fragment is further displaced. Lateral and 45° pronated oblique radiographs usually reveal the dorsal cortical fracture; however, a CT scan may be needed to elucidate body fractures. It is important to inspect the entire wrist, because 12% to 25% of

triquetral injuries are the result of a perilunate fracture dislocation pattern as well as fractures of the radius and ulna [7,8,9,82].

There are two mechanisms by which dorsal cortical fractures occur. Extreme palmar flexion or twisting with avulsion of the fragment by the dorsal radiocarpal and dorsal intercarpal ligaments is one mechanism; however, most injuries are described as hyperextension and ulnar deviation, or fall on outstretched hand (FOOSH). The pathomechanics are believed to involve either a compression effect by the hamate or the ulnar

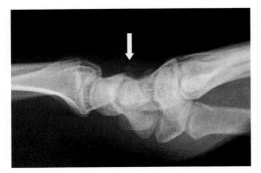

Fig. 8. Triquetrum dorsal cortical fracture (*arrow*), lateral radiograph.

styloid along the dorsum of the triquetrum [83]. A study by Garcia-Elias [84] revealed that in 76 wrists with dorsal cortical fractures, the mean size of the ulnar styloid process was found to be significantly larger than those in a control group of 100 noninjured hands. This study supported the mechanism of the styloid process striking the triquetrum upon extreme wrist dorsiflexion and ulnar deviation causing a dorsal cortical fracture. Compression between the ulna/pisiform and hamate or a direct blow to the triquetrum can result in body fractures. Palmar cortical fractures occur by either avulsion of palmar ulnar triquetral ligament or lunotriquetral ligament, shear from pisiform subluxation, or dislocation.

Treatment for dorsal cortical fractures is a wrist splint or short arm cast for 4 to 6 weeks. According to Hocker and Menschik [83], 86% of patients had a good result after 4-year follow-up, even patients who had up to 4 mm of displacement. Surgery is indicated for persistent symptoms where fragment excision and possible ligament repair are needed. For nondisplaced body fractures, treatment is a short-arm cast for 6 weeks. For a displaced body fracture, closed reduction internal fixation versus ORIF (dorsal approach between the fourth and fifth extensor compartments) is indicated. Treatment of the palmar cortical fracture is closed reduction internal fixation versus ORIF if there is carpal instability secondary to carpus ligamentous avulsion, and excision of fragment and pisiform for a symptomatic pisiform shear injury [85]. Box 5 provides diagnosis and treatment guidelines.

Fractures of the hamate

Fractures of the hamate are divided into body and the more common hook fractures (Fig. 9)

Box 5. Triquetrum summary

Classification [95]
Type 1. Dorsal cortical (Fig. 8)
Type 2. Body
  a. Medial tuberosity
  b. Sagittal
  c. Transverse proximal pole
  d. Transverse body
  e. Comminuted
Type 3. Palmar cortical

Mechanisms
Type 1. (Dorsal cortical fractures)
  - Hyperextension during fall with impaction by ulnar styloid
  - Extreme palmar flexion / twist with avulsion by dorsal ligaments (DRC, DIC)
Type 2. (Body fractures)
  - Direct blow
  - Anteroposterior crush
  - Perilunate injury
Type 3. (Palmar cortical fractures)
  - Avulsion of palmar ligaments
  - Shear from pisiform

Treatment
Type 1.
  - Small fragment, no instability: wrist splint vs. SAC × 4–6 weeks. Excision if symptomatic after 6 months
  - Signs of carpal instability: ORIF
Type 2.
  - Nondisplaced body fracture: SAC × 4–6 weeks
  - Displaced body fracture: CRIF vs ORIF
Type 3.
  - Small fragment, no instability: Wrist splint vs. SAC × 4–6 weeks
  - Ligamentous avulsion with carpal instability: ORIF
  - Shear from pisiform: SAC × 4–6 weeks; excision of fragment and pisiform if remains symptomatic

---

Abbreviations: DIC, dorsal intercarpal ligament; DRC, dorsal radiocarpal ligament.

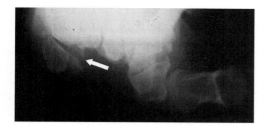

Fig. 9. Hamate hook fracture, base, displaced (*arrow*). Carpal tunnel view radiograph. (Courtesy of Martin A. Posner, MD, New York, NY.)

[86]. Classically, hook of the hamate fractures occur in patients who play racquet sports or golf, with the patient describing pain with gripping activities after the injury. The mechanism of injury is believed to be from repeated microtrauma. On

history, the patient more commonly reports a fall or direct blow to the hand. The examination reveals tenderness over the hypothenar eminence and pain with flexion of the ring and little fingers as the hook acts as a pulley for these tendons [7,8,9,87]. Pain is exacerbated with wrist dorso-ulnar deviation because of fragment movement. The ulnar nerve and artery should be addressed because paresthesias may occur or delayed capillary refill may be encountered. Imaging should include multiple areas with PA, lateral, supinated oblique, and carpal tunnel views. Scheufler and coworkers [87] reported 71% sensitivity when all plain views were considered; however, CT scan offers 100% sensitivity.

The treatment of acute hook fractures is an ulnar gutter short-arm cast for 3 weeks, followed by short-arm cast for 3 weeks. Whalen and colleagues

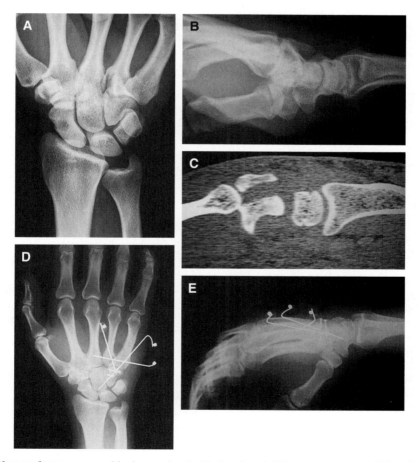

Fig. 10. (*A*) Hamate fracture, coronal body associated with fourth and fifth carpometacarpal dislocations, PA radiograph. (*B*) Lateral radiograph. (*C*) Sagittal CT. (*D*) Open reduction internal fixation, PA radiograph. (*E*) Open reduction internal fixation, oblique radiograph.

[88] demonstrated that acute fractures, when immobilized for 6 weeks, will heal adequately as long as they are minimally displaced. For nonunion, Fujioka and coworkers [89] reported success gaining union with low-intensity pulsed ultrasound. For chronic, symptomatic nonunion, treatment is excision of the fracture fragment. A biomechanical study on cadavers [90] revealed a 15% reduction in grip strength with fragment excision; therefore, patients should be counseled appropriately before surgery. Scheufler and colleagues [87] recently recommended early ORIF or excision for acute hook of hamate fractures, although this remains controversial at this time.

The surgical approach requires an incision over the hypothenar crease. The hamate is positioned between the carpal tunnel and Guyon's canal. The ulnar nerve and artery are decompressed, identified, and protected throughout the procedure. Excision is subperiosteal, which decreases injury to the ulnar motor branch [87].

Nondisplaced, stable body fractures usually heal with immobilization in an ulnar gutter short-arm cast for 3 weeks, followed by short-arm cast for 3 weeks. Surgery is indicated when symptoms persist secondary to nonunion [7,8]. Specific body fractures that involve the proximal wedge (pole) or a coronal pattern require special attention. The wedge (pole) fracture, or fracture to the proximal aspect of the hamate is susceptible for avascular necrosis. The vascularity of this segment relies on an intrinsic osseous blood supply, whereas the distal hamate is perfused both volarly and dorsally by extrinsic sources. Persistent pain and weakness are often the symptoms encountered, and excision of the necrotic segment with hamate to triquetrum fusion may offer relief [91].

Fractures in the coronal plane are usually unstable and require closed reduction internal fixation versus ORIF. The fracture pattern is the result of an axial force by the fourth or fifth metacarpal bones, and often creates carpometacarpal joint instability. Fixation is therefore required to stabilize the joint. Common fixation techniques are pinning and screw fixation (Figs. 10A–E) [92]. Box 6 provides diagnosis and treatment guidelines.

Fractures of the trapezoid

Because of its location, injuries to the trapezoid are rare, accounting for 0.2% of all carpal fractures. Anatomically, the trapezoid is situated in a protected position between the trapezium,

---

Box 6. Hamate summary

Classification [95]
Type 1. Hook (Fig. 9)
  a. Tip (avulsion)
  b. Waist
  c. Base
Type 2. Body
  a. Proximal pole
  b. Medial tuberosity
  c. Sagittal oblique (usually radial to hook)
  d. Coronal (usually with 4/5 CMC fracture dislocation) (Fig. 10)

Mechanisms
Type 1. (Hook)
  - Repeated microtrauma (golf, tennis, etc.) or direct blow
Type 2. (Body)
  a. Wrist fracture-dislocation
  b. Direct blow
  c. AP crush
  d. Axial load of 4th/5th metacarpals

Special Radiographs (CT scan still often necessary)
1. Carpal tunnel view (Fig. 9)
2. Oblique (45° supinated)

Treatment
Type 1. (Hook):
  - Acute: Ulnar gutter cast × 3 weeks, SAC × 3 weeks (controversial: some authors recommend ORIF vs early excision for acute, displaced waist, or base fractures)
  - Chronic, symptomatic nonunion: excision of bony fragment
  - Ulnar nerve/artery symptoms with displaced hook (excision, decompression)
Type 2. (Body):
  - Nondisplaced body: Ulnar gutter cast × 3 weeks, SAC × 3 weeks
  - Displaced body: CRIF vs ORIF (Fig. 10)

Abbreviations: AP, anteroposterior; CMC, carpometacarpal.

Box 7. Trapezoid summary

Classification [95]
Type 1. Dorsal rim
Type 2. Body

Mechanisms
- Axial load of index metacarpal
- Extreme index metacarpal palmar flexion

Treatment
- Nondisplaced: SATSC × 4–6 weeks
- Displaced: CRIF vs ORIF
- Chronic with arthritic changes: CMC arthrodesis

scaphoid, capitate, and second metacarpal bones. It is wedge-shaped; the dorsal facet is twice the size of the palmar facet, which causes fractures and dislocations to displace dorsally when the second metacarpal is driven into extreme flexion [7,9,93]. In addition to the orientation, the palmar ligaments are stronger than its dorsal attachments, and therefore the bone is susceptible to displacement dorsally. The trapezoid is perfused by separate circulations on the volar and dorsal surfaces, where 70% of the blood supply is delivered dorsally. When there is dorsal displacement, the vasculature may be ruptured, predisposing the trapezoid to avascular necrosis [93].

Fracture dislocations are the result of high-energy forces that create multiple injuries. Therefore the metacarpals, as well as the carpal bones, require a thorough inspection during treatment planning. Isolated injuries are caused by extreme palmar flexion by the second metacarpal leading to fracture or dorsal dislocation. Clinically, there is point tenderness at the dorsal trapezoid as well as pain exacerbation with manipulation of the second metacarpal bone. Plain radiographs often do not suffice, and a CT scan is required to make a definitive diagnosis. PA and oblique views may show an empty space with proximal migration of the second metacarpal or dorsal displacement of the trapezoid, respectively [7–9,93,94].

Nondisplaced fractures should be managed nonoperatively with a short-arm thumb spica cast for 4 to 6 weeks. Displaced fractures should be treated with closed reduction internal fixation versus ORIF. Closed reduction may be achieved by distraction of the thumb and second metacarpal as well as palmarly directed pressure over

the dorsal aspect of the trapezoid [93,94]. If closed reduction fails, ORIF is performed through a dorsal incision. Carpometacarpal arthrodesis is reserved for chronic mal- or nonunion with arthritic changes. Box 7 provides diagnosis and treatment guidelines.

Summary

Carpal fractures are uncommon but potentially devastating injuries. Physical examination and standard plain radiographs may reveal only subtle findings. Knowledge of expected fracture patterns and use of special radiographic views or CT scans should aid in making the diagnosis. Nondisplaced fractures should be treated nonoperatively. For intra-articular carpal bone fractures, virtually any amount of displacement is unacceptable and requires reduction and fixation. Depending on the bone, differing blood supply anatomy may play a role in the prognosis of nonunion and risk of AVN. Chronic cases of carpal nonunion, AVN, and arthritis my require salvage procedures of proximal row carpectomy, partial or complete wrist arthrodesis, or arthroplasty.

References

[1] Chung KC, Spilson SV. The frequency and epidemiology of hand and forearm fractures in the United States. J Hand Surg [Am] 2001;26:908–15.

[2] Hove T. Fractures of the hand. Scand J Plast Recons Surg 1993;27(4):317–9.

[3] Van Onselen EB, Karim RB, Hage JJ, et al. Prevalence and distribution of hand fractures. J Hand Surg [Br] 2002;28:491–5.

[4] Shaheen MAE, Badr AA, Al-Khudairy N, et al. Patterns of accidental fractures and dislocations in Saudi Arabia. Injury 1990;1(21):347–50.

[5] Emmet JE, Breck LW. A Review and analysis of 11,000 fractures seen in a private practice of orthopaedic surgery 1937–1956. J Bone Joint Surg [Am] 1958;40:1169–75.

[6] Teisen H, Hjarbaek J. Classification of fresh fractures of the lunate. J Hand Surg [Br] 1988;13: 458–62.

[7] Botte MJ, Gelberman RH. Fractures of the carpus, excluding the scaphoid. Hand Clin 1987;3(1): 149–61.

[8] Bryan RS, Dobyns JH. Fractures of the carpal bones other than lunate and navicular. Clin Orthop 1980; 149:107–11.

[9] Cohen MS. Fractures of the carpal bones. Hand Clin 1997;13(4):587–99.

[10] Rand JA, Linscheid RL, Dobyns JH. Capitate fractures: a long-term follow-up. Clin Orthop 1982;165: 209–16.

[11] Harrigan AH. Fracture of the os magnum. Ann Surg 1908;48(6):917–22.

[12] Adler JB, Shaftan GW. Fractures of the capitate. J Bone Joint Surg [Am] 1962;44:1537–47.

[13] Calandruccio JH, Duncan SFM. Isolated nondisplaced capitate waist fracture diagnosed by magnetic resonance imaging. J Hand Surg [Am] 1999;24: 856–9.

[14] Guiral J, Gracia A, Diaz-Otero JM. Isolated fracture of the capitate with a volar displaced fragment. Acta Orthop Belg 1993;59:406–8 [in French].

[15] Hopkins SR, Ammann W. Isolated fractures of the capitate: use of nuclear medicine as an aid to diagnosis. Int J Sports Med 1990;11:312–4.

[16] Richards RR, Paitich CB, Bell RS. Internal fixation of a capitate fracture with Herbert screws. J Hand Surg [Am] 1990;15:885–7.

[17] Young TB. Isolated fracture of the capitate in a 10-year old boy. Injury 1986;17:133–4.

[18] Enna CD. Isolated pathological fracture of the capitate bone: a case report. Hand 1979;11: 329–31.

[19] Vizkelety T, Wouters HW. Stress fracture of the capitate. Arch Chir Neerl 1972;24:47–57.

[20] Kuniyoshi K, Toh S, Nishikawa S, et al. Long-term follow-up of a malunited isolated fracture of the capitate in a 6-year old boy. J Pediatr Orthop 2005;14B: 46–50.

[21] Thompson NW, O'Donnell M, Thompson NS, et al. Internal fixation of an isolated fracture of the capitate using the Herbert-Whipple screw. Injury 2004; 35(5):541–2.

[22] Yoshihara M, Sakai A, Toba N, et al. Nonunion of the isolated capitate waist fracture. J Orthop Sci 2002;7(5):578–80.

[23] De Schrijver F, De Smet L. Isolated fracture of the capitate: the value of MRI in diagnosis and follow up. Acta Orthop Belg 2002;68(3):310–5 [in French].

[24] Rebuzzi E. Isolated fracture of the capitate with proximal pole dorsal dislocation. A case report. Acta Orthop Belg 2001;67(3):283–5 [in French].

[25] Mikes K. Isolated fracture of the capitate bone. Acta Chir Orthop Traumatol Cech 1964;31:417–21 [in Czech].

[26] Gandolfi M, Zanoli S. The isolated fracture of the capitate eminence. Arch Ortop 1959;72:1485–93 [in Italian].

[27] Mullett H, Shannon F, Syed A, et al. Nonunion of the capitate with associated triangular fibrocartilage tear. Arch Orthop Trauma Surg 2001;121: 362–3.

[28] Rico AA, Holguin PH, Martin JG. Pseudoarthrosis of the capitate. J Hand Surg [Br] 1999;24(3): 382–4.

[29] Gelberman RH, Gross MS. The vascularity of the wrist: identification of arterial patterns at risk. Clin Orthop 1986;202:40–9.

[30] Gelberman RH, Panagis JS, Taleisnik J, et al. The arterial anatomy of the human carpus. Part I: the extraosseous vascularity. J Hand Surg [Am] 1983; 8:367–75.

[31] Panagis JS, Gelberman RH, Taleisnik J, et al. The arterial anatomy of the human carpus. Part II: the intraosseous vascularity. J Hand Surg [Am] 1983;8: 375–82.

[32] Fenton RL, Rosen H. Fractures of the capitate bone. Report of two cases. Bull Hosp Joint Dis 1950;11:134–9.

[33] Minami M, Yamazaki J, Chisaka N, et al. Nonunion of the capitate. J Hand Surg [Am] 1987;12: 1089–91.

[34] Schmitt O, Temme C. Carpaltunnelsyndrome bei Pseudarthrosebildung nach isolierter Fraktur des Os capitatum [Carpal tunnel syndrome in developing pseudarthrosis following isolated fracture of os capitatum]. Arch Orthop Trauma Surg 1978;93: 25–8 [in German].

[35] Grend VR, Dell PC, Glowczewskie F, et al. Intraosseous blood supply of the capitate and its correlation with aseptic necrosis. J Hand Surg [Am] 1984;9: 677–80.

[36] Dahlin LB, Besjakov J. An unusual variant of fracture through the capitate bone—a case report. Acta Orthop Scand 2002;73(2):232–3.

[37] Albertsen J, Mencke S, Christensen L, et al. Isolated capitate fracture diagnosed by computed tomography. Case report. Handchir Mikrochir Plast Chir 1999;31(2):79–81 [in German].

[38] Bretlau T, Christensen OM, Edstrom P, et al. Diagnosis of scaphoid fracture and dedicated extremity MRI. Acta Orthop Scand 1999;70(5):504–8.

[39] Rayan GM. Occult wrist pain due to capitate nonunion. South Med J 1994;87(3):402–4.

[40] Schick S, Trattnig S, Gabler C. Okkulte Handgelenkfrakturen: Feinfokusvergrosserungsrontren versus MRT [Occult fractures of the wrist joint: high resolution image magnification roentgen versus MRI]. Rofo 1999;170(1):16–21 [in German].

[41] Volk AG, Schnall SB, Merkle P, et al. Unusual capitate fracture: a case report. J Hand Surg [Am] 1995; 20:581–2.

[42] Heim U. Pseudarthrose des Kapitatums [Pseudarthrosis of the capitate]. Handchirurgie 1986;18:158–60 [in German].

[43] Lowry WE Jr, Cord SA. Traumatic avascular necrosis of the capitate bone—case report. J Hand Surg [Am] 1981;6:245–8.

[44] Fleege MA, Jebson PJ, Renfrew DL, et al. Pisiform fractures. Skeletal Radiol 1991;20:169–72.

[45] Palmieri TJ. Pisiform area pain treatment by pisiform excision. J Hand Surg [Am] 1982;7:477–80.

[46] Marti T, Gimilio GG. Study of the isolated fracture of the pisiform bone. Schweiz Rundsch Med Prax 1973;62:968–9 [in French].

[47] Vasilas A, Grieco VR, Bartone NF. Roentgen aspects of injuries to the pisiform bone and

pisotriquetral joint. J Bone Joint Surg [Am] 1960; 42:1317–28.

[48] Carroll RE, Coyle MP Jr. Dysfunction of the pisotriquetral joint: treatment by excision of the pisiform. J Hand Surg [Am] 1985;10:703–7.

[49] Israeli A, Engel J, Ganel A. Possible fatigue fracture of the pisiform bone in volleyball players. Int J Sports Med 1982;3:56–7.

[50] Turecki E. Isolated fracture of the pisiform bone. Chir Narzadow Ruchu Ortop Pol 1972;37:17–9 [in Polish].

[51] Dufek P, Thormahlen F, Ostendorf U. Fracture of the pisiform bone in inline skating. Sportverletz Sportschaden 1999;13(2):59–61 [in German].

[52] Cavlak Y. Fracture of the pisiform bone. Aktuelle Traumatol 1994;24(2):68–9 [in German].

[53] Lacey JD, Hodge JC. Pisiform and hamulus fractures: easily missed wrist fractures diagnosed on a reverse oblique radiograph. J Emerg Med 1998;16: 445–52.

[54] Abbit PL, Riddervold HO. The carpal tunnel view: helpful adjuvant for unrecognized fractures of the carpus. Skeletal Radiol 1987;16(1):45–7.

[55] Failla JM, Amadio PC. Recognition and treatment of uncommon carpal fractures. Hand Clin 1988;4: 469–76.

[56] Matsunaga D, Uchiyama S, Nakagawa H, et al. Lower ulnar nerve palsy related to fracture of the pisiform bone in patients with multiple injuries. J Trauma 2002;53:364–8.

[57] Howard FM. Ulnar-nerve palsy in wrist fractures. J Bone Joint Surg 1961;43:1197–201.

[58] Georgoulis A, Hertel P, Lais E. Fracture and dislocation fracture of the os pisiforme. Unfallchirurg 1991;94(4):182–5 [in German].

[59] Rettig ME, Dassa GL, Raskin KB, et al. Wrist fractures in the athlete. Distal radius and carpal fractures. Clin Sports Med 1998;17(3):469–89.

[60] Geissler WB. Carpal fractures in athletes. Clin Sports Med 2001;20(1):167–88.

[61] Muniz AE. Unusual wrist pain: pisiform dislocation and fracture. J Emerg Med 1999;17:78–9.

[62] Palmieri TJ. The excision of painful pisiform bone fractures. Orthop Rev 1982;11:99–103.

[63] Razemon JP. Fractures of the carpal bones. In: Tubiana R, editor. The hand, vol. II. Philadelphia: WB Saunders; 1985. p. 821–43.

[64] Borgeskov S, Christiansen B, Kjaer A, et al. Fractures of the carpal bones. Acta Orthop Scand 1966; 37:276–87.

[65] Cooney WP III, Chao EYS. Biomechanical analysis of static forces in the thumb during hand function. J Bone Joint Surg [Am] 1977;59:27–36.

[66] Inston N, Pimpalnerkar AL, Arafa MAM. Isolated fracture of the trapezium: an easily missed injury. Injury 1997;28(7):485–8.

[67] McGuigan FX, Culp RW. Surgical treatment of intra-articular fractures of the trapezium. J Hand Surg [Am] 2002;27:697–703.

[68] Cordrey LJ, Ferrer-Torells M. Management of fractures of the greater multangular. J Bone Joint Surg [Am] 1960;42:1111–8.

[69] Palmer AK. Trapezial ridge fractures. J Hand Surg [Am] 1981;6:561–4.

[70] Freeland AE, Finley JS. Displaced vertical fracture of the trapezium treated with a small cancellous lag screw. J Hand Surg [Am] 1984;9:843–5.

[71] Jones WA, Ghorbal MS. Fractures of the trapezium —a report on three cases. J Hand Surg [Br] 1985;10: 227–30.

[72] Jones JA, Pellegrini VD. Transverse fracture-dislocation of the trapezium. J Hand Surg [Am] 1989; 14:481–5.

[73] Horch R. A new method for treating isolated fractures of the os trapezium. Acta Orthop Trauma Surg 1998;117:180–2.

[74] Taleisnik J. The wrist. New York: Churchill Livingston; 1985.

[75] Garavaglia G, Bianchi S, Santa DD, et al. Trans-trapezium carpo-metacarpal dislocation of the thumb. Arch Orthop Trauma Surg 2004; 124:67–8.

[76] Foster RJ, Hastings H II. Treatment of Bennett, Rolando, and vertical intraarticular trapezial fractures. Clin Orthop 1987;214:121–9.

[77] Walker JL, Greene TL, Lunseth PA. Fractures of the body of the trapezium. J Orthop Trauma 1988; 2:22–8.

[78] Pointu J, Schwenck JP, Destree G, et al. Fractures of the trapezium. Mechanisms. Anatomo-pathology and therapeutic indications. Rev Chir Orthop Reparatrice Appar Mot 1988;74(5):454–65 [in French].

[79] Gelberman RH, Vance RM, Zakaib GS. Fractures at the base of the thumb: treatment with oblique traction. J Bone Joint Surg [Am] 1979; 61:260–2.

[80] Freeland AE, Ahmad N. Oblique shear fractures of the lunate. Orthopedics 2003;26(8):805–8.

[81] Gelberman RH, Bauman TD, Menon J, et al. The vascularity of the lunate bone and Kienbock's disease. J Hand Surg [Am] 1980;5:272–8.

[82] De Beer JD, Hudson DA. Fractures of the triquetrum. J Hand Surg [Br] 1987;12:52–3.

[83] Hocker K, Menschik A. Chip fractures of the triquetrum. Mechanism, classification and results. J Hand Surg [Br] 1994;19:584–8.

[84] Garcia-Elias M. Dorsal fractures of the triquetrum —avulsion or compression fractures? J Hand Surg [Am] 1987;12:266–8.

[85] Suzuki T, Nakatsuchi Y, Tateiwa, et al. Osteochondral fracture of the triquetrum: a case report. J Hand Surg [Am] 2002;27:98–100.

[86] Milch H. Fracture of the hamate bone. J Bone Joint Surg [Am] 1932;16:459–62.

[87] Scheufler O, Andresen R, Radmer S, et al. Hook of hamate fractures: critical evaluation of different therapeutic procedures. Plast Reconst Surg 2005; 115(2):488–97.

[88] Whalen JL, Bishop AT, Linsheid RL. Nonoperative treatment of acute hamate hook fractures. J Hand Surg [Am] 1992;17:507–11.

[89] Fujioka H, Tsunoda M, Noda M, et al. Treatment of ununited fracture of the hook of hamate by low-intensity pulsed ultrasound: a case report. J Hand Surg [Am] 2000;25:77–9.

[90] Demirkan F, Calandruccio JH, Diangelo D. Biomechanical evaluation of flexor tendon function after hamate hook excision. J Hand Surg [Am] 2003;28: 138–43.

[91] Van Demark RE, Parke WW. Avascular necrosis of the hamate: a case report with reference to the hamate blood supply. J Hand Surg [Am] 1992;17: 1086–90.

[92] Ebraheim NA, Skie MC, Savolaine ER, et al. Coronal fracture of the body of the hamate. J Trauma 1995;38(2):169–74.

[93] Cuenod P, Della Santa DR. Open dislocation of the trapezoid. J Hand Surg [Br] 1995;20:185–8.

[94] Miyawaki T, Kobayashi M, Matsuura S, et al. Trapezoid bone fracture. Ann Plast Surg 2000;44:444–6.

[95] Putnam MD, Meyer NJ. Carpal fractures excluding the scaphoid. In: Trumble TE, editor. Hand surgery update 3. Rosemont (IL): American Society for Surgery of the Hand; 2003. p. 175–87.

ELSEVIER
SAUNDERS

Hand Clin 22 (2006) 517–528

HAND
CLINICS

Carpal Osteoarthrosis

Brett Peterson, MD, Robert M. Szabo, MD, MPH*

*Department of Orthopaedic Surgery, University of California Davis School of Medicine, 4860 Y Street,
Suite 3800 Sacramento, CA 95817, USA*

Despite improved understanding of carpal mechanics, increased awareness of intercarpal ligament injuries, and improved techniques for treating carpal instability, post-traumatic intercarpal osteoarthrosis remains a common problem. Osteoarthritis of the carpal bones, including scapholunate advance collapse (SLAC) wrist, scaphotrapeziotrapezoid (STT) arthritis, lunotriquetral arthritis, triquetrohamate arthritis, and pisotriquetral arthritis, follows specific unique patterns, but in each, the final common pathway leads to degenerative change. Injury or deformity leads to instability and altered kinematics producing abnormal joint contact pressures. Cartilage injury and eventual degeneration of the joint follow. The etiology, prevalence, and current evaluation and treatment of these conditions is of importance to hand surgeons.

Scapholunate advanced collapse and scaphoid nonunion advanced collapse wrist

Scapholunate instability and collapse is by far the most frequent cause of noninflammatory degenerative arthritis of the wrist [1,2]. With a fall on an outstretched hand, the wrist moves into dorsiflexion, ulnar deviation, and supination. The first structure injured is the scapholunate interosseous ligament; with greater force, the radioscaphocapitate, long radiolunate, and dorsal radiocarpal ligaments may be torn [3–5]. This progression of injury, described by Mayfield [3], can be seen radiographically as scapholunate

dissociation, triquetrolunate dissociation, and finally perilunate and lunate dislocation. With disruption of the scapholunate interosseous ligament, the scaphoid assumes a more flexed position; the capitate is able to move proximally, and the lunate, its connection to the triquetrum maintained, assumes a more dorsiflexed position. This pattern of carpal collapse or instability is described as dorsiflexion intercalary segment instability (DISI) (Fig. 1) [6].

Because of the particular geometry of the scaphoid and distal radius articular surfaces, stress risers develop at abnormal contact points of the articular surface. With time, the abnormal stresses lead to degeneration of the articular cartilage, and a typical pattern of arthritic change develops. The cascade of degenerative change begins with radioscaphoid arthritis, followed by capitolunate and scaphotrapeziotrapezoid arthritis. Ultimately, pan-wrist arthritis results [7,8]. As Watson and Ballet [1] described, the SLAC wrist pattern is classified into four stages . In Stage I, increased contact pressures lead to beaking of the radial styloid. Narrowing and arthrosis of the radioscaphoid joint indicates progression to Stage II. In Stage III, arthrosis develops between the capitate and the scaphoid or the lunate. There is also proximal migration of the capitate. Finally, at Stage IV, all of the previous stage changes occur, along with degeneration of the radiolunate joint. When arthrosis is limited to the radial styloid, reconstructive procedures of the scapholunate ligament, along with styloid excision, are the treatment of choice [9]. When there is arthrosis of the radioscaphoid joint (Stage II) or Stage III with additional arthrosis in the midcarpal joint, scapholunate ligament reconstructive procedures are no longer indicated. Stage II disease salvage

---

* Corresponding author.

E-mail address: rmszabo@ucdavis.edu
(R.M. Szabo).

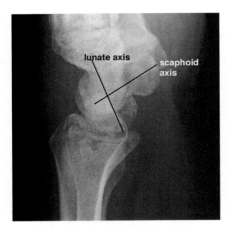

Fig. 1. Lateral view of the wrist in a patient with a chronic scapholunate injury. In the radiograph, scaphoid and lunate axes are drawn in. There is an increased scapholunate angle and the wrist shows a DISI pattern.

procedures such as four-corner fusion or proximal row carpectomy (PRC) preserve wrist motion and are preferable to total wrist fusion [10,11]. If the proximal capitate is arthritic, a PRC is contraindicated unless a soft tissue arthroplasty as described by Eaton [12] is added, and a four-bone fusion procedure is favored [13]. Total wrist fusion is the standard treatment for Stage IV disease, although arthroplasty remains an option in selected patients.

Scaphoid nonunion advanced collapse (SNAC) wrist is analogous to the more common SLAC wrist [14]. The natural history of scaphoid nonunion is one of progressive wrist arthritis [15,16]. In a retrospective review of 102 patients who had scaphoid nonunions, Inoue and Sakuma [17] found that the prevalence of arthritis was 22% in nonunions of less than 5 years duration, 75% in nonunions of 5 to 9 years duration, and 100% in nonunions of 10 years or more duration. Arthritic changes initially appear at the radioscaphoid joint as radial styloid beaking and dorsal scaphoid osteophyte formation. Later changes include arthritis of the radioscaphoid, midcarpal arthritis, and finally pan-wrist arthritis. This pattern is very similar to that of the development of SLAC wrist, although with SNAC wrist, the radial fossa that articulates with the proximal pole of the scaphoid escapes degenerative changes until late in the disease process. The prevalence of a DISI deformity increases with time after nonunion [18]. The four stages of progression of SNAC wrist are similar to the patterns seen with SLAC wrist, as have been described [1].

Clinical examination

After obtaining a complete history of the patient's previous injuries, including location, duration, work history, aggravating factors, previous treatments, and job status, it is important to search for potential systemic causes of arthritis. Crystalline arthropathy or rheumatoid disease may cause an SLAC wrist pattern that may also involve the radiolunate joint [19,20]. Physical examination should include palpation for areas of maximal tenderness, which is actually one of the most useful tools for diagnosis of patients who have chronic wrist problems [21,22]. Areas to palpate include the scapholunate ligament area, STT joint, and the radial border of the scaphoid. Range of motion, grip strength, and neurovascular status should also be assessed, and if indicated, appropriate provocative tests such as the scaphoid shift test are performed. It is important to note if a particular range of motion produces pain. For example, pain in radial deviation is common with early SLAC and SNAC wrist.

Radiographic evaluation

The initial radiographic evaluation should include at least four views of the wrist. These include a posteroanterior (PA) view, a lateral view, a clenched-fist ulnar deviation PA (scaphoid) view, and a 45° semipronated view. The PA view should be done with the patient's elbow flexed to 90° and the shoulder abducted 90°, with the forearm in neutral rotation (ulnar variance view). In the PA view without radial or ulnar deviation, Gilula's lines can be drawn and should be smooth. In addition, an abnormal outline of the lunate on the PA view may indicate a DISI or volar intercalated segment instability (VISI) deformity [23]. The PA radiograph of a wrist with a DISI deformity shows the lunate with a wedge-shaped ulnar corner pointing toward the medial side of the wrist, whereas radiographs of a VISI deformity wrist tend to show the lunate with a C-shaped outline. The lateral of the wrist must be a true lateral, with the wrist in neutral rotation. In the true lateral view, the pisiform lies between the scaphoid tuberosity and the capitate head [24]. The semipronated view places the dorsoulnar and radiopalmar portions of the wrist in profile. Additional views such as an AP clenched-fist view may help to assess the radiocarpal joint, the midcarpal joint, and the relationship of the scaphoid to the lunate (Fig. 2).

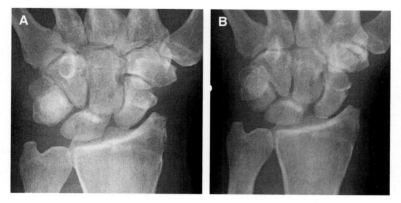

Fig. 2. (*A*) PA radiograph of patient with complaint of dorsal wrist pain. (*B*) Same patient with a clenched fist view.

Treatment

The treatment of SLAC wrist is controversial. Earlier stages of scapholunate dissociation may be treated with a combination of ligament repair and dorsal intercarpal ligament capsulodesis. Reported results of series by Blatt [25], Wyrick and colleagues [26], Szabo and coworkers [27], and Wintman and coworkers [28], indicate improvements in alignment and pain, although there is concern of these results diminishing with time. When diagnosis of the scapholunate ligament injury is delayed, the exact chronicity of the problem may be difficult to determine. Therefore, choosing the best surgical treatment option may be challenging, especially in cases of carpal collapse in combination with beginning osteoarthrosis of the radial styloid and the proximal pole of the scaphoid (Fig. 3). Wieloch and colleagues [29] reported on eight patients who had Stage I SLAC wrist and underwent scapholunate ligament reconstruction. This was performed on average 66 months after the initial injury. At 2 years, five of eight patients reported wrist improvement after the scapholunate ligament reconstruction; however, three of eight patients reported worsening wrist symptoms. All of the patients had abnormal carpal height ratios, both pre- and postoperatively and at follow-up. The study authors' conclusions were that scapholunate dissociation with early stages of arthritis remains an unsolved problem [29]. In a survey of American and Canadian hand surgeons, Zarkadas and colleagues [30] noted that, although there was a consensus on the treatment of early scapholunate ligament injuries, the treatment of chronic injuries was highly variable.

For Stage II disease, traditionally, a four-bone fusion (capitate, hamate, lunate, triquetrum) along with scaphoid excision was recommended for active patients. PRC was reserved for patients who had lower demands and who were also less tolerant of a longer period of immobilization [31]. There has not been a randomized study comparing these two operations, but Cohen and Kozin [32] reported results of PRC versus four-corner fusion in two comparable groups of patients. In the study, two cohorts of patients from separate institutions performing exclusively either a scaphoid excision and four-corner arthrodesis or PRC for SLAC wrist were compared. In both groups, there were 19 patients who were comparable with respect to age, gender, dominance, stage of arthritis, or preoperative measures of pain and function. The length of the follow-up period averaged 28 months for the four-corner arthrodesis group and 19 months for the PRC patients. At follow-up, there were no significant differences in the wrist flexion-extension arc, averaging 81° in the PRC patients and 80° following four-corner arthrodesis. Grip strength of the affected hand compared with the opposite hand averaged 71% for the PRC group compared with 79% for the four-corner arthrodesis patients.

Recently, Baumeister and colleagues [33] reported on a series of 38 patients who had Stage II disease—SNAC-wrist (n = 29) or SLAC-wrist (n = 9). Postoperative examination included range of motion and grip strength. Mean extension and flexion of the wrist reached 75°, which was 57% of that of the contralateral hand. Mean radial and ulnar deviation was 33°, compared with 52% of that of the contralateral hand. The average grip

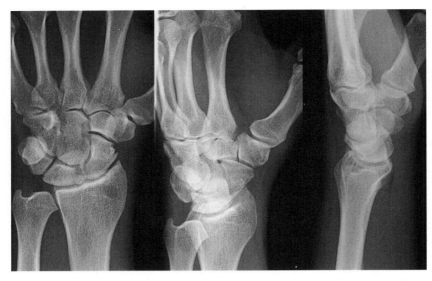

Fig. 3. 45-year-old patient with chronic scapholunate dissociation. The patient shows signs of an early scapholunate advanced collapse. The lateral radiograph (far right) shows DISI pattern, and degenerative changes are seen at the radioscaphoid articulation.

strength was 50% of the unaffected side. Pain with strenuous activity was reduced by 40%, and resting pain was reduced by 77%. Three patients showed radiological signs of a radiocapitate arthrosis. One patient needed conversion to a complete wrist arthrodesis. These results were noted at an average of 27 months after surgery, and were in agreement with the rest of the literature; however, consistent with other reviews of proximal row carpectomy, the long-term results are not known. In a separate study, Dacho and colleagues [13] reviewed their results in 49 patients at 47 months after midcarpal arthrodesis [33]. Active range of motion was 56% of that of the nonoperated wrist and grip strength was 76%. Forty-five patients demonstrated bony consolidation; however, 6 patients needed further treatment with a total wrist arthrodesis because of pain or absence of bony consolidation. Overall, 77% of the patients returned to their original occupation, and 80% were satisfied with the final result.

Both PRC and scaphoid excision with four-corner arthrodesis are motion-preserving options for the treatment of SLAC arthritis, with minimal subjective or objective differences in short-term follow-up evaluations. Scaphoid excision and four-corner fusion is indicated in more severe disease, and appears to offer the potential for longer durability; however, there is little objective evidence to support this assertion (Fig. 4).

For early SNAC wrist, Soejima and coworkers [34] reported on a series of 9 patients in whom excision of the distal pole of the scaphoid gave good results at an average of 28.6 month follow-up. Before surgery, all patients had recalcitrant scaphoid nonunions and associated degenerative arthritis. Patients underwent excision of the distal scaphoid fragment. At an average of 28.6 months follow-up, wrist range of motion had improved from 51.4% to 94% of that of the opposite wrist. Grip strength improved from 40% to 77% of that of the opposite wrist. Based on a modified Mayo wrist scoring chart, clinical results were excellent in 6 patients and good in 3. Eight patients showed no radiographic progression of arthritis, whereas one patient who had a Type II lunate (facet articulation with hamate [35]) did progress to arthritis. Malerich and colleagues [18] reported on a series of 19 patients who underwent distal scaphoid excision for degenerative arthritis secondary to scaphoid nonunion. They also noted improvement in pain, grip strength, and range of motion with this procedure, although they cautioned that in patients who had capitolunate arthritis, symptoms tended to persist and degenerative changes progressed. Overall the results are encouraging for a procedure that is simpler and requires less immobilization than a four-corner fusion, at least in patients who had no capitolunate arthritis.

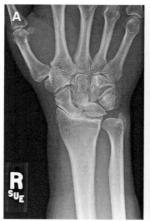
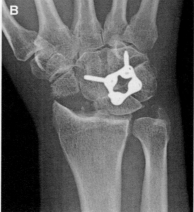

Fig. 4. (*A*) Patient with Stage III SLAC wist including capitolunate arthritis. (*B*) After partial scaphoid excision and four-corner fusion.

Lunotriquetral arthritis

Although degenerative problems associated with scapholunate dissociation are a very common cause of wrist arthritis, isolated lunotriquetral arthritis is rare unless it is encountered as a result of a partial carpal coalition [36]. Coalition of carpal bones is relatively common, and the lunate-triquetrum fusion is the most frequent carpal coalition [36,37]. This finding is almost always coincidental and asymptomatic (Fig. 5); however, when the coalition is incomplete, patients who have this problem may have ulnar-sided wrist pain [38] and arthritic changes in the remaining lunotriquetral joint.

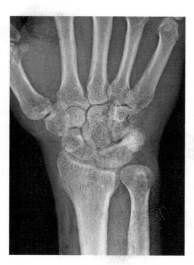

Fig. 5. Patient with an isolated lunotriquetral coalition. Patient was asymptomatic from the coalition.

Clinical and radiologic evaluation

It is important to differentiate isolated lunotriquetral problems from other causes of ulnar sided wrist pain such as triangular fibrocartilage complex (TFCC) tears. After a complete physical examination, standard radiographs are obtained. There must be a true lateral radiograph to rule out a VISI deformity and a zero-rotation PA radiograph to assess ulnar variance. An arthrogram or magnetic resonance arthrogram may be a useful study because it is not uncommon to see TFCC and lunotriquetral pathology together.

Treatment

As discussed earlier, isolated lunotriquetral arthritis is rare unless it is the result of a partial carpal coalition. This is one of the few clear indications for isolated lunotriquetral arthrodesis. Treatment of ligamentous injuries to the lunotriquetral articulation is more controversial.

Lunotriquetral ligament injuries may result in a VISI deformity. For a VISI pattern to develop, there must be disruption of the dorsal and palmar lunotriquetral ligaments as well as the dorsal radiotriquetral and dorsal radioscaphotriquetral ligaments [39]. Unotriquetral fusion or ligament reconstruction is recommended only if there is isolated lunotriquetral instability without a VISI deformity [40,41]. In addition, nonunion rates of lunotriquetral fusion are higher if the patient has positive ulnar variance. If there is a VISI deformity, isolated lunotriquetral arthrodesis is contraindicated, because the static deformity will not be corrected. The hamate must be included in the lunotriquetral fusion or a four-bone fusion must be performed. If there is positive ulnar variance along with an isolated lunotriquetral ligament injury or lunotriquetral arthritis, the positive variance should be corrected at the time of lunotriquetral fusion.

Kirschenbaum and colleagues [42] reported on a series of lunotriquetral fusions in 14 patients. All patients had chronic LT instability and underwent lunotriquetral fusion. The follow-up period averaged 27 months. Radiographs were suggestive of fusion in 12 of the cases. One of the pseudarthroses required revision surgery, the other was asymptomatic. One patient had persistent wrist pain. Wrist motion compared with the contralateral side averaged 85%, 88%, 83% and 80%, respectively, for flexion, extension, ulnar deviation, and radial deviation. Grip strength compared with the contralateral side averaged 93%. The study authors concluded that LT fusion reliably relieves pain while maintaining functional wrist motion and grip strength [42].

Scaphotrapeziotrapezoid osteoarthritis

Isolated STT arthritis is less common than SLAC patterns of arthritis [43,44], and the etiology of STT arthritis is not as well understood. In Watson and Ballet's paper [1], SLAC wrist accounted for 57% of arthritic wrists, whereas 27% of cases occurred between the scaphoid, trapezium, and trapezoid; a combination of these two patterns occurred in 15% [1]. Previous studies have associated STT arthritis with isolated scapholunate ligament disruption [35]. Cope [45] demonstrated in a cadaveric study that abnormal scaphoid rotation, rotatory subluxation of the scaphoid, is prevented if the scaphotrapezial and radiocarpal ligaments are intact, even if the scapholunate interosseous ligament is disrupted. With disruption of all of these ligaments, the resulting rotatory subluxation of the scaphoid leads to abnormal pressures on the radioscaphoid articulation and eventual arthritis of the radiocarpal joint [45]. Consistent with this concept of isolated scapholunate ligament injury leading to STT arthritis, Viegas and coworkers [35] noted that isolated STT arthritis was associated with an increased scapholunate interval, but not with a ring sign or radiocarpal arthritis. Presumably, these patients had isolated scapholunate ligament injury that led to the STT arthritis, but because the other ligaments were intact, there was no rotatory subluxation of the scaphoid or development of radiocarpal arthritis and the SLAC wrist pattern.

More recently, a study examining radiographs of 1711 patients visiting an emergency room in the United Kingdom were reviewed over a 5-month period [46]. Isolated STT arthritis was seen in 1% of the population, was predominantly in females, and was often asymptomatic [46]. The study authors found that the majority of patients who had STT arthritis did not have scapholunate ligament disruption, thus contesting the notion that isolated scapholunate ligament injury leads to STT arthritis. Instead, it was suggested that general degenerative disease accounted for the association between STT arthritis and isolated scapholunate ligament tears.

Clinical and radiologic evaluation

The initial evaluation of STT arthritis is similar to that of patients who have SLAC wrist. In patients who have STT arthritis, swelling and fullness will be noted in the anatomic snuffbox and volar radial wrist. Volar pressure on the scaphoid or flexor carpi radialis tunnel will elicit tenderness, which is exacerbated by radial deviation and gripping. Additional radiographic views include a hyperpronated view of the wrist, which may show early changes in the STT joint. These views will also allow assessment of the first carpometacarpal (CMC) joint (Fig. 6). Severe CMC arthritis can lead to involvement of the STT joint; however, the treatment of pan-trapezial arthritis differs from that of isolated STT arthritis and is not discussed here.

Treatment

For patients who have symptomatic STT arthritis that is refractory to conservative treatment, surgical options include arthroscopic debridement, resection arthroplasty, or STT fusion. Ashwood and coworkers [47] have reported success with arthroscopic debridement for isolated STT arthritis, although this procedure is controversial. Ten patients who had persistent symptoms underwent arthroscopic debridement of the STT joint. Nine patients reported good or excellent results at an average follow-up of 36 months; however, as with arthroscopy for other arthritic joints, debridement offers at best only temporary relief. Most clinicians prefer STT fusion.

Reported results from STT fusion vary. Meier and colleagues [48] reported on 111 patients who

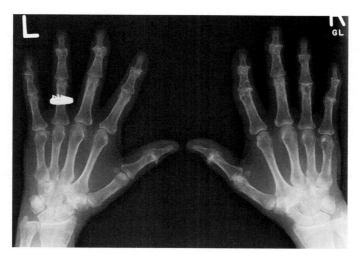

Fig. 6. Bilateral AP views of the hands in a patient with radial sided wrist pain. Patient has osteoarthritis of the distal interphalangeal (DIP) joints as well as bilateral STT arthritis.

were treated with STT fusion from 1992 to 1997. Indications were chronic dissociation of the scapholunate joint (n = 15), idiopathic arthrosis of the scaphotrapeziotrapezoid joint (n = 11), Kienbock's disease in advanced stage (n = 84), and dislocation of the trapezium (n = 1). After an average follow-up period of 4 years (range 2 to 8 years), patients showed an average wrist motion in extension and flexion of 81% of the preoperative range, and in radial and ulnar deviation of 68% of the preoperative range. Preoperative pain values were reduced. The average grip strength improved to 65% of the contralateral side. Good results were reached according to the modified Mayo wrist score, with a score of 66 points (71 points in arthritis of the STT joint, 62 points in Kienbock's disease, 60 points in SL-dissociation). The patients described low disability in the Disabilities of the Arm, Shoulder and Hand (DASH) scores, with an average of 27 points. At 4 years, the data showed that STT fusion was reliable and effective for treatment and pain relief, and offers reasonable functional results [48].

Unfortunately, although several operations may be effective at limiting rotatory subluxation of the scaphoid, few operations are able to correct scapholunate gap. This applies to both ligamentous reconstructions and to scaphotrapeziotrapezoid fusion. STT/triscaphe fusion is used to stabilize the radial column of the wrist. Kleinman and colleagues [49] analyzed the effects of STT arthrodesis on wrist kinematics in a series of patients. They followed 41 patients who underwent

STT fusion: 25 patients had chronic static scapholunate instability and 16 patients had dynamic instability. The average follow up was 56 months. Postoperative planar radiographs and cineradiographic examination in patients were performed. Scapholunate diastasis that was present before the operation persisted after the operation. This was noted with in ulnar deviation of the wrist. In ulnar deviation, the STT fusion mass, capitate, and hamate rotate with the hand while the lunate-triquetral unit is not physiologically "pulled" radially into the lunate fossa of the radius.

Alternatives to STT fusion include resection arthroplasty as well as pyrocarbon implants. Garcia-Elias and coworkers [50] reviewed a series of 21 patients who underwent distal scaphoid excision for STT arthritis. In some of the surgeries, the defect was filled with capsular or tendinous tissue, and in approximately half, the defect was not filled. Thirteen of the wrists were pain-free and 8 reported mild discomfort at an average follow-up of 29 months. Grip strength, pinch strength, and motion improved, and 15 patients returned to their previous jobs. The 6 patients who were previously unemployed reported no limitations in activities. In the past, there has been little success with prosthetic replacements for intercarpal osteoarthritis, although Pequignot and colleagues [51] recently reported on treating STT arthritis using a pyrocarbon implant. Fifteen cases that occurred between 1994 and 2002 were reviewed, with an average follow-up of 4 years. The study authors reported improvements in pain and grip strength, and stressed that this intervention restored mobility without the destabilization of carpal bones seen with distal scaphoid excision. In addition, they reported a low complication rate for a procedure that could be later revised to an STT fusion if necessary [51].

Pisotriquetral arthritis

Chronic pain in the pisiform area may be caused by tendinitis of the insertion of the flexor carpi ulnaris, bony fractures, or osteoarthrosis of the pisotriquetral joint, which some report as a frequent site of osteoarthritis slightly less common than the scaphotrapezial osteoarthrosis [52]. Although pain and tenderness on the palmar and ulnar aspects of the wrist in the area of the pisiform bone is fairly common, refractory pisotriquetral osteoarthritis was unusual enough for Green to be able to make a case report of simple excision of the pisiform back in 1979 [53]. Subperiosteal excision of pisiform bone is customarily performed after unsuccessful initial nonoperative treatment, and although the postoperative results seem to be rather good, Beckers and Koebke [54] have recently reported on some functional limitations resulting from pisiform excision.

Clinical and radiologic evaluation

Osteoarthritis of the pisotriquetral joint is most often caused by acute and chronic trauma and instability. The symptoms of osteoarthritis of the pisotriquetral joint are pain over the pisiform, with pressure and grinding of the joint. There may be ulnar nerve symptoms, and attrition or rupture of the flexor profundus tendon to the little finger. Based on the history, physical examination, and radiographic findings, osteoarthritis of the pisotriquetral joint must be differentiated from extensor carpi ulnaris tendinitis, TFCC disorders, lunotriquetral disorders, and flexor carpi ulnaris tendinitis. The best radiographic view to evaluate the pisotriquetral joint is the supinated oblique view (Fig. 7). This view is obtained by having the patient position both hands palm up on the radiographic plate, as though he were holding a large bowl.

Treatment

Conservative treatment of pisotriquetral arthritis consists of local injections of steroid into the pisotriquetral joint along with nonsteroidal anti-inflammatory drugs (NSAIDs) and protective splinting. When conservative therapy fails, consideration should be given to pisiform excision.

Review of the literature on pisotriquetral arthritis reveals several small case series that report good results with pisiform excision. Gomez and colleagues [55] retrospectively reviewed and reported on 21 patients with a mean age of 42 who were treated with excision of the pisiform for a dysfunction of the pisotriquetral joint. The diagnoses included degenerative arthritis of the pisotriquetral joint (15 patients), degenerative arthritis associated with a ganglion (3 patients), and calcifications caused by flexor carpi ulnaris tendinopathy (3 patients). All patients had pain secondary to direct pressure on the pisiform. Side-to-side passive motion of the pisiform occasionally led to pain and crepitus. Degenerative arthritis and calcifications in the pisotriquetral joint were confirmed by a wrist radiograph. In 5 patients, local injection with anesthetic temporarily resolved the symptoms. At an average of 30 months follow-up, excision of the pisiform was reported as giving excellent pain relief with no functional losses.

A recent study by Gaston and coworkers [56] focused on pisotriquetral arthritis after midcarpal fusion. Their study was a retrospective review of nine patients requiring pisiform excision after wrist or inter-carpal arthrodesis. Six patients underwent four-corner fusions and three underwent wrist fusion. On average, patients presented with ulnar-sided wrist pain at 15 months after surgery. After other causes of pain were ruled out, all nine patients underwent pisiform excision with resolution of symptoms. In the second part of the study, a cadaver model was used to analyze the kinematics and pressure of the pisotriquetral joint for various wrist intercarpal fusion positions. The cadaveric study revealed that maximum pisotriquetral pressures occurred at full dorsiflexion and progressively decreased with flexion. Gaston and colleagues concluded that the pisotriquetral joint should be assessed before midcarpal fusion or total wrist fusion, and highlighted performing the fusion in the appropriate amount of extension [56].

Despite the excellent results reported in these clinical studies, Beckers and Koebke [54] have reported on potential instability after pisiform excision. In their anatomic study of 112 pisotriquetral joints, mechanical tests were performed to investigate the distribution of forces within the pisiform and the pisotriquetral joint. The study authors found that the pisiform contributes to the stability

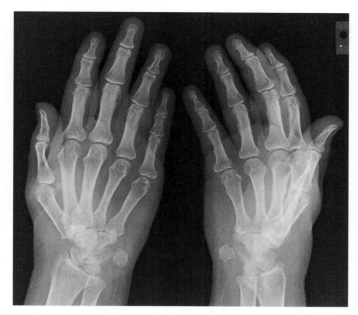

Fig. 7. Supinated oblique view of 49-year-old patient with bilateral ulnar-sided wrist pain. Patient has bilateral pisotriquetral arthritis. PA views of wrists appeared normal.

of the ulnar column by supporting the triquetrum in extension and as a fulcrum for transferring forearm muscle forces to the wrist. When the pisiform was excised, this resulted in what they termed "microinstability" in their cadaver model [54]. Whether this microinstability will translate into clinical symptoms remains to be determined.

Carpal boss

Multiple descriptions and case reports of carpal boss exist in the literature [57–60]. A carpal boss may be confused with a ganglion or an accessory bone such as an accessory capitate [61]; however, a true carpal boss is a bony protuberance on the dorsum of the wrist at the base of the second and third metacarpals. It may be a degenerative osteophyte or an accessory ossification center known as an os styloideum. This ossicle is thought to develop early in embryogenesis, and trivial injury to this area may induce degenerative changes; often the condition is seen in younger patients.

Clinical and radiographic evaluation

When a carpal boss is symptomatic, patients complain of pain and limitation of motion. The symptoms may result from an overlying bursitis, an extensor tendon slipping over the bony prominence, a ganglion, or arthritic changes at this site.

After the history and physical examination, it is important to obtain a full radiographic series to characterize and locate the lesion. Radiographically, the view that best profiles the separate os styloideum is a lateral view using 30° of supination and ulnar deviation of the wrist (Fig. 8) [62].

Treatment

Symptomatic carpal boss typically responds to anti-inflammatory medication, splinting, and corticosteroid injection. If these conservative measures fail, the anatomic abnormality may be excised. Most reports note that simple excision gives excellent relief, but that for more pronounced degenerative changes, carpometacarpal fusion may be necessary [60,63–66]. Fusi and co-workers [65] reviewed their results of surgical treatment of carpal boss. They treated 116 patients with an average age of 32 years. The localized bony abnormality and the associated degenerative arthritic process were resected back to normal articular surface and normal adjacent cancellous bone. At a mean follow-up of 42 months, complete symptomatic relief was observed in 94% of the patients. Recurrence or persistence of symptoms developed in seven patients. Six had a second operation, and all of these patients reported relief of symptoms [65]. In another series of 44 patients followed over a period of 7 years

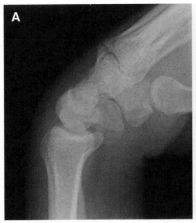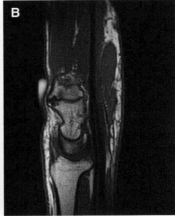

Fig. 8. 31-year-old male with a dorsal bony prominence at base of third metacarpal. Lateral radiograph (*A*) and MRI (*B*) show the carpal boss at the capitate-third metacarpal joint.

[64], 21 patients underwent surgery using a similar technique. Overall results were good, with no recurrence of deformity, although 2 patients complained of pain with strenuous activities. In contrast, Clarke and coworkers [66] reviewed 48 patients who had symptomatic carpal boss seen during a 10-year period. Thirty-one patients had undergone either local excision or arthrodesis of the affected carpometacarpal joint. Mean follow-up was 3 years. Nine cases had to be revised, and 24 patients remained symptomatic and considered their surgery a failure. These remarkably contrasting results by Clarke and colleagues [66] versus those by Fusi and coworkers [65] bring the comparability of their study groups into question, and provide yet another example of the need for prospective studies that comprehensively assess patient symptoms and function.

Summary

Despite improved understanding of carpal mechanics, increased awareness of intercarpal ligament injuries, and improved techniques for treating carpal instability, post-traumatic intercarpal osteoarthrosis remains a common problem. The authors have focused on specific patterns and regions of carpal osteoarthritis. When symptomatic treatments such as splinting, local injections, and anti-inflammatory medications fail, surgical intervention becomes an option. The surgical options of excision or limited fusion have limitations and potential complications. These operations must be critically evaluated to determine which are most effective. Even limited excisions such as of the pisiform, as suggested by Beckers and Koebke [54], may have significant functional consequences; however, when successful, these operations can provide pain relief, restore wrist stability, and improve function [7].

Acknowledgments

The authors wish to thank Dr. John C. Hunter for his assistance in providing clinical radiographs.

References

[1] Watson HK, Ballet FL. The SLAC wrist: scapholunate advanced collapse pattern of degenerative arthritis. J Hand Surg [Am] 1984;9(3):358–65.

[2] Mack GR, Bosse MJ, Gelberman RH, et al. The natural history of scaphoid non-union. J Bone Joint Surg Am 1984;66(4):504–9.

[3] Mayfield JK. Patterns of injury to carpal ligaments. A spectrum. Clin Orthop Relat Res 1984;187:36–42.

[4] Mayfield JK. Wrist ligamentous anatomy and pathogenesis of carpal instability. Orthop Clin North Am 1984;15(2):209–16.

[5] Mayfield JK. Mechanism of carpal injuries. Clin Orthop Relat Res 1980;149:45–54.

[6] Watson HK, Black DM. Instabilities of the wrist. Hand Clin 1987;3(1):103–11.

[7] Watson HK, Ryu J. Evolution of arthritis of the wrist. Clin Orthop Relat Res 1986;202:57–67.

[8] Krimmer H, Krapohl B, Sauerbier M, et al. Post-traumatic carpal collapse (SLAC- and SNAC-wrist)—stage classification and therapeutic

possibilities. Handchir Mikrochir Plast Chir 1997; 29(5):228–33 [in German].

[9] Allende BT. Osteoarthritis of the wrist secondary to non-union of the scaphoid. Int Orthop 1988;12(3): 201–11.

[10] Krakauer JD, Bishop AT, Cooney WP. Surgical treatment of scapholunate advanced collapse. J Hand Surg [Am] 1994;19(5):751–9.

[11] Krimmer H, Sauerbier M, Vispo-Seara JL, et al. Advanced carpal collapse (SLAC-wrist) in scaphoid pseudarthrosis. Therapy concept: medio-carpal partial arthrodesis. Handchir Mikrochir Plast Chir 1992;24(4):191–8 [in German].

[12] Eaton RG. Proximal row carpectomy and soft tissue interposition arthroplasty. Tech Hand Up Extrem Surg 1997;1(4):248–54.

[13] Dacho A, Grundel J, Harth A, et al. Functional outcome after midcarpal arthrodesis in the treatment of advanced carpal collapse (SNAC-/SLAC-wrist). Handchir Mikrochir Plast Chir 2005;37(2):119–25 [in German].

[14] Sauerbier M, Bickert B, Trankle M, et al. Surgical treatment possibilities of advanced carpal collapse (SNAC/SLAC wrist). Unfallchirurg 2000;103(7): 564–71 [in German].

[15] Ruby LK, Leslie BM. Wrist arthritis associated with scaphoid nonunion. Hand Clin 1987;3(4):529–39.

[16] Osterman AL, Mikulics M. Scaphoid nonunion. Hand Clin 1988;4(3):437–55.

[17] Inoue G, Sakuma M. The natural history of scaphoid non-union. Radiographical and clinical analysis in 102 cases. Arch Orthop Trauma Surg 1996;115(1): 1–4.

[18] Malerich MM, Clifford J, Eaton B, et al. Distal scaphoid resection arthroplasty for the treatment of degenerative arthritis secondary to scaphoid nonunion. J Hand Surg [Am] 1999;24(6):1196–205.

[19] Berger RA, Buckwalter JA. Calcium pyrophosphate dihydrate crystal deposition patterns in the triangular fibrocartilage complex. Orthopedics 1990;13(1): 75–80.

[20] Cleak DK. Dislocation of the scaphoid and lunate bones without fracture: a case report. Injury 1982; 14(3):278–81.

[21] Chidgey LK. Chronic wrist pain. Orthop Clin North Am 1992;23(1):49–64.

[22] Taleisnik J. Pain on the ulnar side of the wrist. Hand Clin 1987;3(1):51–68.

[23] Cantor RM, Braunstein EM. Diagnosis of dorsal and palmar rotation of the lunate on a frontal radiograph. J Hand Surg [Am] 1988;13(2):187–93.

[24] Yang Z, Mann FA, Gilula LA, et al. Scaphopisocapitate alignment: criterion to establish a neutral lateral view of the wrist. Radiology 1997;205(3): 865–9.

[25] Blatt G. Capsulodesis in reconstructive hand surgery. Dorsal capsulodesis for the unstable scaphoid and volar capsulodesis following excision of the distal ulna. Hand Clin 1987;3(1):81–102.

[26] Wyrick JD, Youse BD, Kiefhaber TR. Scapholunate ligament repair and capsulodesis for the treatment of static scapholunate dissociation. J Hand Surg [Br] 1998;23(6):776–80.

[27] Szabo RM, Slater RR Jr, Palumbo CF, et al. Dorsal intercarpal ligament capsulodesis for chronic, static scapholunate dissociation: clinical results. J Hand Surg [Am] 2002;27(6):978–84.

[28] Wintman BI, Gelberman RH, Katz JN. Dynamic scapholunate instability: results of operative treatment with dorsal capsulodesis. J Hand Surg [Am] 1995;20(6):971–9.

[29] Wieloch PT, Martini AK, Daecke W. Results of ligament reconstruction in advanced scapholunate dissociation. Handchir Mikrochir Plast Chir 2005; 37(2):90–6 [in German].

[30] Zarkadas PC, Gropper PT, White NJ, et al. A survey of the surgical management of acute and chronic scapholunate instability. J Hand Surg [Am] 2004;29(5): 848–57.

[31] Wyrick JD. Proximal row carpectomy and intercarpal arthrodesis for the management of wrist arthritis. J Am Acad Orthop Surg 2003;11(4):277–81.

[32] Cohen MS, Kozin SH. Degenerative arthritis of the wrist: proximal row carpectomy versus scaphoid excision and four-corner arthrodesis. J Hand Surg [Am] 2001;26(1):94–104.

[33] Baumeister S, Germann G, Dragu A, et al. Functional results after proximal row carpectomy (PRC) in patients with SNAC-/SLAC-wrist Stage II. Handchir Mikrochir Plast Chir 2005;37(2): 106–12 [in German].

[34] Soejima O, Iida H, Hanamura T, et al. Resection of the distal pole of the scaphoid for scaphoid nonunion with radioscaphoid and intercarpal arthritis. J Hand Surg [Am] 2003;28(4):591–6.

[35] Viegas SF, Patterson RM, Hokanson JA, et al. Wrist anatomy: incidence, distribution, and correlation of anatomic variations, tears, and arthrosis. J Hand Surg [Am] 1993;18(3):463–75.

[36] Simmons BP, McKenzie WD. Symptomatic carpal coalition. J Hand Surg [Am] 1985;10(2):190–3.

[37] Delaney TJ, Eswar S. Carpal coalitions. J Hand Surg [Am] 1992;17(1):28–31.

[38] Ritt MJ, Maas M, Bos KE. Minnaar type 1 symptomatic lunotriquetral coalition: a report of nine patients. J Hand Surg [Am] 2001;26(2):261–70.

[39] Horii E, Garcia-Elias M, An KN, et al. A kinematic study of luno-triquetral dissociations. J Hand Surg [Am] 1991;16(2):355–62.

[40] Lichtman DM, Noble WH 3rd, Alexander CE. Dynamic triquetrolunate instability: case report. J Hand Surg [Am] 1984;9(2):185–8.

[41] Guidera PM, Watson HK, Dwyer TA, et al. Lunotriquetral arthrodesis using cancellous bone graft. J Hand Surg [Am] 2001;26(3):422–7.

[42] Kirschenbaum D, Coyle MP, Leddy JP. Chronic lunotriquetral instability: diagnosis and treatment. J Hand Surg [Am] 1993;18(6):1107–12.

[43] Wilhelm K, Rolle A, Hild A. The scaphoid-trapezium-trapezoid arthrosis. A clinical study 1982–1985. Unfallchirurg 1989;92(2):59–63 [in German].

[44] Moritomo H, Viegas SF, Nakamura K, et al. The scaphotrapezio-trapezoidal joint. Part 1: An anatomic and radiographic study. J Hand Surg [Am] 2000;25(5):899–910.

[45] Cope JR. Rotatory subluxation of the scaphoid. Clin Radiol 1984;35(6):495–501.

[46] Higginson AP, Braybrook J, Williams S, et al. Isolated scaphotrapeziotrapezoid osteoarthritis: prevalence, symptomatology and associated scapholunate ligament disruption in a population presenting to an accident and emergency department with acute wrist injuries. Clin Radiol 2001;56(5):372–4.

[47] Ashwood N, Bain GI, Fogg Q. Results of arthroscopic debridement for isolated scaphotrapeziotrapezoid arthritis. J Hand Surg [Am] 2003;28(5):729–32.

[48] Meier R, Prommersberger KJ, Krimmer H. Scaphotrapezio-trapezoid arthrodesis (triscaphe arthrodesis). Handchir Mikrochir Plast Chir 2003;35(5):323–7 [in German].

[49] Kleinman WB. Long-term study of chronic scapholunate instability treated by scapho-trapezio-trapezoid arthrodesis. J Hand Surg [Am] 1989;14(3):429–45.

[50] Garcia-Elias M, Lluch AL, Farreres A, et al. Resection of the distal scaphoid for scaphotrapeziotrapezoid osteoarthritis. J Hand Surg [Br] 1999;24(4):448–52.

[51] Pequignot JP, D'Asnieres de Veigy L, Allieu Y. Arthroplasty for scaphotrapeziotrapezoidal arthrosis using a pyrolytic carbon implant. Preliminary results. Chir Main 2005;24(3–4):148–52 [in French].

[52] Fischer E. Pisotriquetral arthrosis and the so-called pisiform secundarium. Radiologe 1988;28(7):338–44 [in German].

[53] Green DP. Pisotriquetral arthritis: a case report. J Hand Surg [Am] 1979;4(5):465–7.

[54] Beckers A, Koebke J. Mechanical strain at the pisotriquetral joint. Clin Anat 1998;11(5):320–6.

[55] Gomez CL, Renart IP, Pujals JI, et al. Dysfunction of the pisotriquetral joint: degenerative arthritis treated by excision of the pisiform. Orthopedics 2005;28(4):405–8.

[56] Gaston GRLG, Floyd WE, Swick M. Pisotriquetral arthritis following wrist and inter-carpal arthrodesis. Paper presented at the 23rd Annual Adrian E Flatt Residents and Fellows Conference in Hand Surgery. September, 2005.

[57] Alverno L, Repossi G. Considerations on 7 cases of carpal boss. Pathologica 1960;52:45–52 [in Italian].

[58] Dorosin N, Davis JG. Carpal boss. Radiology 1956; 66(2):234–6.

[59] Cuono CB, Watson HK. The carpal boss: surgical treatment and etiological considerations. Plast Reconstr Surg 1979;63(1):88–93.

[60] van der Aa JP, Noorda RJ, van Royen BJ. Symptomatic carpal boss. Orthopedics 1999;22(7):703–4.

[61] Tielliu IF, van Wellen PA. Carpal boss caused by an accessory capitate. Case report. Acta Orthop Belg 1998;64(1):107–8 [in French].

[62] Conway WF, Destouet JM, Gilula LA, et al. The carpal boss: an overview of radiographic evaluation. Radiology 1985;156(1):29–31.

[63] Hazlett JW. The third metacarpal boss. Int Orthop 1992;16(4):369–71.

[64] Lenoble E, Foucher G. The carpal bump. Ann Chir Main Memb Super 1992;11(1):46–50 [in French].

[65] Fusi S, Watson HK, Cuono CB. The carpal boss. A 20-year review of operative management. J Hand Surg [Br] 1995;20(3):405–8.

[66] Clarke AM, Wheen DJ, Visvanathan S, et al. The symptomatic carpal boss. Is simple excision enough? J Hand Surg [Br] 1999;24(5):591–5.

Wrist Arthrofibrosis

Steve K. Lee, MD[a],*, Francesco Gargano, MD[b],
Michael R. Hausman, MD[b]

[a]New York University Hospital for Joint Diseases Orthopaedics Institute, The New York
University School of Medicine, 301 East 17th Street, New York, NY 10003, USA
[b]Department of Orthopaedic Surgery, The Mount Sinai School of Medicine, 5 East 98th Street,
Box 1188, New York, NY 10029, USA

Motion-limiting arthrofibrosis has been described in numerous joints, including the knee [1–4], ankle [5,6], shoulder [7–10], and elbow [11,12]. Clinically, arthrofibrosis is characterized by limited joint motion and pain [13]. Although less well described, arthrofibrosis also occurs in the wrist joint [14,15]. The normal range of motion of the wrist is 70 degrees of extension and 80 degrees of flexion, 30 degrees of ulnar and 20 degrees of radial deviation, 80 degrees of pronation and 80 degrees of supination [16]. However, less than half of total wrist motion permits almost all of functional range of motion. Palmer and associates [17] determined that functional ranges of wrist motion for most activities of daily living are 5 degrees of flexion, 30 degrees of extension, 10 degrees of radial deviation, and 15 degrees of ulnar deviation, and Morrey and associates [18] determined that forearm rotation of 50 degrees of supination and 50 degrees of pronation was necessary for most activities. More recent studies have reported that most activities could be performed with 40 degrees of wrist flexion and extension, 10 degrees radial deviation, and 30 degrees ulnar deviation [19,20]. Arthrofibrosis is characterized by pain and limitation of motion beyond that required for most daily activities, as defined above.

Etiology and pathophysiology

Stiffness and decreased range of motion are common following trauma or surgery to the wrist. This usually resolves with physiotherapy. Arthrofibrosis is defined as pain and stiffness that does not allow functional range of motion and is due to adhesions or contracture of the joint. The etiology of contracture of a joint can be classified into either intraarticular or extraarticular [21]. Arthrofibrosis is due to an excessive fibrotic response during the repair process, which leads to fibrotic tissue deposition, within or around the joint, and progressive loss of motion of the joint [22].

The mechanism is initiated by an excessive synovial inflammatory response with activation and proliferation of fibroblast cells and a significant increase in the deposition of extracellular matrix proteins [23,24]. It is believed that the pathophysiology first involves inflammation of the synovium, then subsynovial fibrosis, leading to capsular thickening, and ultimately contracture of the affected joint [9,23–26].

Although the etiology is still unknown, there are alterations of the extracellular matrix with an increase of collagen type VI expression similar to other local or systemic fibrotic disorders [27]. A chronic inflammatory process may play a crucial role in the mechanism of primary arthrofibrosis, and may indicate an immune response [28]. Association with human leukocyte antigens and dysregulation of cytokine release have been demonstrated to be involved in its pathogenesis [29–32].

No benefits in any form have been received or will be received from a commercial party related directly or indirectly to the subject of this article.

* Corresponding author.

E-mail address: steve.lee@nyumc.org (S.K. Lee).

Clinical manifestations

The clinical diagnosis of arthrofibrosis is often one of exclusion. Classic symptoms appear after surgery or trauma, especially after prolonged period of immobilization of greater than 6 weeks. The disorder is characterized by a limitation of both active and passive range of motion of the wrist joint that is not primarily due to arthritis or other underlying conditions. Swelling and pain are invariably accompanying symptoms, and often lead to sleep disturbance.

Despite intensive physiotherapy, the wrist range of motion does not achieve the expected improvements and a plateau is eventually reached. The progression of the disability leads to stiffness and restricted movement. Wrist range of motion of flexion-extension, pronation-supination, radial-ulnar deviation, will be variably affected.

Diagnosis

Clinical symptoms of pain, restricted wrist range of motion, swelling, and a plateau in the improvements after at least 6 months of intensive physiotherapy should be considered suspicious for arthrofibrosis. There is frequently a hard endpoint to range of motion.

Before a diagnosis of arthrofibrosis can be made, other causes of loss of motion and pain must be ruled out in the differential diagnosis. This includes bony incongruity, arthritis, complex regional pain syndrome, carpal instability, loose bodies, malunion, nonunion, avascular necrosis, soft tissue (tendons, skin) contracture, spasticity, and skin or subcutaneous scarring. Loss of motion and pain are more commonly caused by one of these entities, and not arthrofibrosis.

The evaluation begins with a thorough history and physical examination. Particular parts of the physical examination include a detailed account of wrist range of motion: flexion, extension, radial deviation, ulnar deviation, supination, and pronation. The quality of endpoints (hard versus soft) and whether there is pain at the endpoints, should be noted. Anesthetic block of the posterior interosseous nerve, anterior interosseous nerve, and distal radioulnar joint with a local anesthetic agent, or examination under anesthesia, can help determine if the limited range of motion is due to pain or structural mechanical pathology.

Wrist radiographs should be evaluated for bony incongruity, arthritis, malunion, nonunion, loose bodies, and carpal instability patterns. If there is a question of bony pathology, which is equivocally seen on radiographs, CT may help elucidate the diagnosis. Dynamic radiographic sequences or fluoroscopy can be useful to assess the motion of the radiocarpal and midcarpal joints in flexion, extension, ulnar, and radial deviation. MRI may be helpful to confirm or deny suspicions of intraarticular fibrous adhesions, ligament injury, or avascular necrosis. Special MRI cartilage sequences with 3D gradient and echo (fat saturated) or fat saturated proton density are taken in coronal or sagittal planes to assess the cartilage status. These studies can also demonstrate capsular thickening.

Classification system

For optimal treatment and planning, we have classified wrist arthrofibrosis based on location of disease and functional limitation (Box 1).

Treatment

Nonoperative

The most common cause of arthrofibrosis is traumatic injury. Therefore, the first step in treatment is prevention. Because protein-rich edema fluid is eventually replaced by scar tissue, edema control is paramount in prevention. This is achieved by strict elevation, compression, and finger exercises.

Once the diagnosis of arthrofibrosis has been made, treatment starts with a dedicated program of therapy to stretch scar tissue. In addition to active, active-assist, and passive range of motion exercises, dynamic and static-progressive splinting regimens may be employed [33–35]. Dynamic splinting is the use of traction devices, such as rubber bands, which produces plastic deformation

---

Box 1. Wrist arthrofibrosis classification

Type I: Intrinsic (adhesions)
   A. Radiocarpal joint (Fig. 1)
   B. Midcarpal joint
   C. Distal radioulnar joint (DRUJ)
   D. Combination of above

Type II: Extrinsic (capsular fibrosis)
   A. Dorsal
   B. Palmar
   C. Distal radioulnar joint (DRUJ)
   D. Combination of above

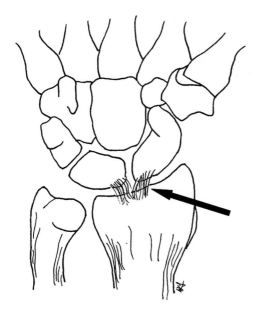

Fig. 1. Fibrous bands (*arrow*) extend from the radius to the carpus (Type IA wrist arthrofibrosis). This "spot welds" the carpus to the radius.

through creep, or the permanent deformation of tissue when placed under constant stress for an extended period of time. Typical dynamic splinting regimens require 8 to 12 hours of splint usage per day. Static-progressive splinting produces plastic deformation through stress–relaxation, or the permanent deformation of tissue when held in a constant deformation. Both methods improve motion of contracted joints, but static-progressive splints require shorter treatment times and are generally better tolerated by patients [33,35].

Most cases do respond to nonoperative treatment. If after 3 months of noninvasive treatment, range of motion remains unacceptable, then intraarticular corticosteroid injection may be indicated, based on data from adhesive capsulitis of the shoulder [36]. If the range of motion has plateaued after 6 months of physiotherapy, splinting, and corticosteroid injections, and the range of motion is inadequate for activities of daily living, surgical treatment may be indicated.

Operative

Types IA, B, and D have intraarticular adhesions (Fig. 1) and are best approached arthroscopically. Surgical arthroscopic treatment of arthrofibrosis has been successfully used for contracture of the knee, shoulder, and elbow [1,3,

9–12,37–39]. Hattori and colleagues [40] have recently reported on arthroscopic treatment of wrist intraarticular adhesions. In a series of 11 patients, they attained improvement in 91% of patients with an average increase of 22 degrees of range of motion.

Arthroscopic radiocarpal and midcarpal joint intrinsic adhesion release

Standard wrist portals are initially used (3–4, 4–5, 6R, 6U, MCR, MCU) and thorough resection of intraarticular adhesions is performed. A combination of shaver, thermal ablation, arthroscopic biters, and graspers are employed. Both radiocarpal and midcarpal joints are inspected and pathologic adhesions debrided. Additional 1-2 and palmar radial portals may be used to visualize and resect adhesions in the dorsal aspect of the joint. The palmar radial portal is made by making a 2-cm incision over the flexor carpi radialis (FCR) tendon at the level of the radiocarpal joint. The tendon sheath is incised and the FCR tendon is retracted ulnarly. The portal is made through the FCR subsheath [41].

Types IC and II C are best approached by the open procedure as described by Kleinman and Graham [42,43] (Fig. 2). Open dorsal and palmar capsulectomies of the distal radioulnar joint have been described by the authors for posttraumatic contracture of the distal radioulnar joint capsule limiting supination and pronation. They reported on nine patients who had average gains of 51 degrees of supination from 21 degrees preoperatively to 72 degrees postoperatively and 28 degrees of pronation gain from 54 degrees preoperatively to 82 degrees postoperatively [42].

Open distal radioulnar joint contracture release (Kleinman and Graham technique)

Palmar distal radioulnar joint release

Palmar capsulectomy is indicated for loss of supination [42]. It is performed by approaching the DRUJ through an interval between the ulnar neurovascular bundle and the flexor carpi ulnaris tendon. The neurovascular bundle is gently retracted ulnarly and the extrinsic flexor muscle mass is retracted radially. The space between the proximal aspect of the palmar radioulnar ligament and distal ulnar head is identified with an 18-gauge needle, which may be confirmed radiographically. The DRUJ arthrotomy is initiated

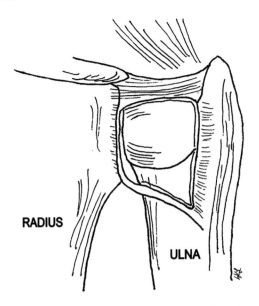

RADIUS

ULNA

Fig. 2. DRUJ "silhouette" capsulectomy. The palmar side is similar. Dorsal and palmar capsulectomies are performed by excising a portion of capsule "silhouetting" the ulnar head. The resection of the central portion of the thickened capsule preserves the critical ligamentous portions of the triangular fibrocartilage complex. (*Adapted from* Kaplan FTD. Stiffness and joint contracture. In: Friedman SL, editor. Complications in orthopaedics—distal radius fractures. Rosemont (IL): American Academy of Orthopaedic Surgeons; 2005. p. 53.)

with a transverse incision in this space. All the elements of the triangular fibrocartilage complex are spared. Complete excision of the palmar capsule is accomplished by first dissecting toward its insertion on the radius, paralleling the proximal margin of the palmar radioulnar ligament. The dissection continues proximally along the margin of the sigmoid notch of the radius to the edge of the proximal aspect of the ulnar head. The scalpel is then directed ulnarward, outlining the hyaline cartilage surface of the palmar aspect of the ulnar head. By following the contour of the distal ulna in this manner, a palmar "silhouette " resection of the DRUJ capsule is accomplished to completely excise the thickened elements of the capsule while protecting the articular surfaces of the distal ulna and distal radial sigmoid notch.

Dorsal distal radioulnar joint release

Dorsal DRUJ capsulectomy is indicated for loss of pronation. The capsule is approached by retracting the extensor digiti quinti from the fifth

dorsal compartment. The floor of the fifth compartment either can be elevated from the underlying dorsal DRUJ capsule or can be included in the silhouette capsulectomy, which is preferable for surgical efficiency. Like the palmar procedure, the space between the proximal aspect of the dorsal radioulnar ligament and the distal ulnar head is identified with an 18-gauge needle. A transverse incision is then made in this space toward the radius, remaining parallel to the distal radioulnar ligament. Incise proximally along the border of the sigmoid notch to the proximal aspect of the ulnar head. Then incise ulnarly, outlining the ulnar head to make a window in the dorsal capsule, which "silhouettes" the ulnar head (Fig. 2). The stout inferior aspect of the capsule is maintained in all cases. Once either the palmar or dorsal capsular resection is performed, any intraarticular adhesions can be lysed with a Freer elevator.

Types IIA, B and D usually do not require surgery; if they do, both open [14] and arthroscopic [44] methods have been described. Watson and Weinzweig [14], using both open dorsal and palmar approaches, have described surgical release of extrinsic joint contracture.

Open wrist extrinsic contracture release (Watson and Weinzweig technique)

For contracture limiting wrist flexion, the dorsum of the wrist is approached through a longitudinal or transverse incision at the level of the radial styloid; it is rarely necessary to completely open any of the extensor retinacular compartments [14]. The tendons are retracted to provide exposure of the wrist joint and dorsal capsulotomy is performed, releasing the dorsal capsule radial to Lister's tubercle and the dorsal radiocarpal ligament (dorsal radiolunotriquetral ligament), which is originates ulnar to Lister's tubercle (Fig. 3). Following release, it is important to analyze wrist motion by fluoroscopy. If the wrist is hinging open dorsally and the radiocarpal motion is not congruous, then a palmar approach is needed to release the proximal row and allow translation until flexion occurs while maintaining normal articular contact. Combined denervation of the posterior interosseous nerve (PIN) and anterior interosseous nerve (AIN) may be performed at the same time to augment pain relief.

For contracture limiting wrist extension or for incongruous radiocarpal motion, a palmar

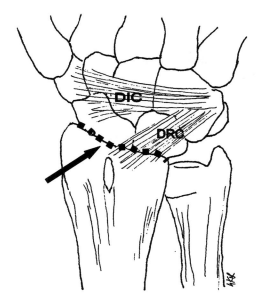

Fig. 3. Dorsal extrinsic release of the radiocarpal joint. Dorsal capsule is incised radial to Lister's tubercle. The dorsal radiocarpal ligament (DRC) is incised ulnar to Lister's tubercle. DIC, dorsal intercarpal ligament. Arrow and dashed line = incision. (*Adapted from* Kaplan FTD. Stiffness and joint contracture. In: Friedman SL, editor. Complications in orthopaedics—distal radius fractures. Rosemont (IL): American Academy of Orthopaedic Surgeons; 2005. p. 53.)

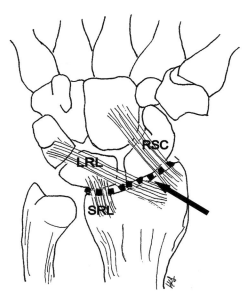

Fig. 4. Palmar extrinsic release of the radiocarpal joint. Scar tissue is incised (*arrow* and *dashed line*), which lies superficial to the important palmar wrist ligaments: radioscaphocapitate (RSC), long radiolunate (LRL), and short radiolunate (SRL). These ligaments are preserved in the open palmar release as proposed by Watson and Weinzweig.

approach is performed through an extended carpal tunnel incision with a 45 degree zig zag incision across the proximal wrist crease in line with the ulnar aspect of the palmaris longus, avoiding injury to the palmar cutaneous branch of the median nerve. The flexor tendon mass and median nerve are gently retracted radially and the ulnar neurovascular bundle is gently retracted ulnarly. The radiocarpal joint line is then identified and motion-limiting scar tissue is incised. This scar tissue lies superficial to the important palmar wrist ligaments, the radioscaphocapitate, long radiolunate (radiolunotriquetral), and short radiolunate ligaments (Fig. 4). The offending scar tissue tends to run longitudinally where the important palmar ligaments run obliquely. The palmar ligaments should be preserved if possible. Intraoperative gains in range of motion should be documented.

Studies on cadavers have demonstrated the safety of arthroscopic capsular release in the shoulder [39] and more recently in the wrist [44]. Verhellen and Bain [44] described arthroscopic

wrist capsular release. This relatively radical release should be approached with caution, because there is one single report of two cases of its use and no other verifying studies. Verhellen and Bain base their technique on the work of Viegas and colleagues [45], who demonstrated in a cadaveric study, that sectioning of numerous ligaments (Fig. 5) did not result in ulnar or palmar translation. With the addition of ulnar carpal (UC) sectioning palmar translation of the carpus occurred. The addition of sectioning of the dorsal ulnar (DUL) and palmar ulnar (PUL) ligaments led to ulnar translation as well. However, there were pressure centroid shifts in the palmar direction of both the scaphoid and lunate when only two ligaments, radioscaphocapitate (RSC) and long radiolunate (LRL) ligaments, were sectioned. It is unclear how this would affect carpal wear patterns in vivo.

Verhellen and Bain [44] performed an anatomic study on 10 MRIs and two cadaveric specimens and reported that the average distance from the radiocarpal joint capsule to the neurovascular structures were 6.9 mm to the median nerve, 6.7 mm to the ulnar nerve, and 5.2 mm to the radial

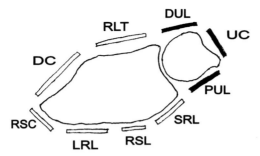

Fig. 5. Ligaments resected in the arthroscopic capsular release as proposed by Verhellen and Bain. Ulnar ligaments (depicted in *black*) should not be sectioned (DUL, UC, PUL) to prevent instability. DC, dorsal capsule; RLT, radiolunotriquetral; DRC, dorsal radiocarpal; DUL, dorsal ulnar; UC, ulnocarpal; PUL, palmar ulnar; SRL, short radiolunate; RSL, radioscapholunate; LRL, long radiolunate; RSC, radioscaphocapitate. (*Redrawn from* Verhellen R, Bain GI. Arthroscopic ·capsular release for contracture of the wrist: a new technique. Arthroscopy 2000;16:108; with permission.)

artery. Distances to the closer tendon structures were not reported. They reported on two cases with average improvements in range of motion of 30 degrees of flexion and 40 degrees extension. There was no clinical or radiographic evidence of carpal instability postoperatively in either case.

Arthroscopic extrinsic wrist contracture release (Verhellen and Bain technique, modified)

The arthroscope is placed in the three to 3-4 and an arthroscopic, hooked electrocautery device is introduced into the working portals of 6R and 4-5 to cut the palmar capsule and ligaments. The ligaments are cut until extracarpal fat and the flexor carpi radialis tendon are visualized. Division of the palmar capsule includes the short radiolunate ligament, the radioscapholunate ligament, the long radiolunate ligament, and the radioscaphocapitate ligament. The ulnotriquetral and ulnolunate ligament are left intact. The dorsal capsule and dorsal radiocarpal (dorsal radiolunotriquetral) ligament is then divided from the sigmoid notch to the radial styloid with the hooked electrocautery device. The dorsal ulnar ligament complex is left intact. The 1-2 and palmar radial portals are useful to visualize and work on dorsal aspects of the radiocarpal joint. The final ligamentous transections are depicted

(Fig. 5). The arthroscopic instruments are removed and gentle closed manipulation is performed to achieve maximal improvement in range of motion, which is documented.

Postoperative treatment

The postoperative treatment should consist of full, unrestricted mobilization of the wrist. Postoperative pain relief is generally well controlled with a wrist block or pain pump indwelling catheter regional block using 0.5% bupivacaine in the immediate postoperative period, followed by oral analgesics. Intensive physiotherapy and splinting should be used to maintain range of motion gained intraoperatively.

Illustrative case

A 22-year-old woman injured her left wrist in a motor vehicle collision (Fig. 6A,B). The fracture was fixed by open reduction internal fixation with a palmar fixed-angle plate and DRUJ pinning (Fig. 7A,B). The fracture healed, but despite 9 months of intensive postoperative physical therapy, the patient developed a painful left wrist and restricted range of motion to 10 degrees of extension and 30 degrees of flexion (Fig. 8A,B). Supination was minimally affected with lack of 10 degrees versus the contralateral side. Pronation, radial, and ulnar deviations were symmetric. Standard radiographs showed good reduction and complete healing of the fracture. MRI showed multiple adhesive fibrous bands from the distal radius to the carpus, which were tethering motion (Fig. 9).

The patient was diagnosed with Type IA wrist arthrofibrosis that had failed nonoperative treatment. Arthroscopy confirmed intraarticular radiocarpal adhesions (Fig. 10). Arthroscopic resection of the adhesions was performed through standard portals (Fig. 11). Postoperative range of motion improved to 70 degrees of extension (increase of 700%) and 80 degrees of flexion (increase of 267%) (Fig. 12A,B). Grip strength improved from 15 kg preoperatively to 50 kg postoperatively (increase of 333%).

Discussion

Arthrofibrosis is an acknowledged cause of pain, limited motion, and disability in multiple joints, including the knee, ankle, shoulder, and

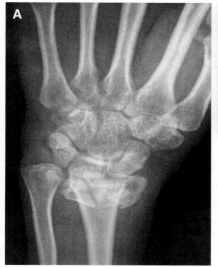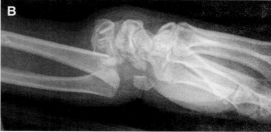

Fig. 6. Preoperative injury films of a severely comminuted distal radius fracture with DRUJ instability. (*A*) Posteroanterior wrist radiograph. (*B*) Lateral wrist radiograph.

elbow [1–12]. Theoretically, no diarthrodial joint is immune from this poorly understood pathologic process, and its incidence in the wrist may be greater than realized [14,15].

Stiffness of the wrist had previously been attributed to capsular thickening and contracture, although evidence to support this conclusion is limited [44]. Intraarticular adhesions characteristic of arthrofibrosis have been observed and reported, but the true incidence is unknown. MRI, especially scans obtained using special cartilage-imaging sequences, may demonstrate intraarticular bands or adhesions. The sensitivity of MRI is, however, unknown and a negative scan does not necessarily exclude arthrofibrosis. Cine fluoroscopy examination may provide additional

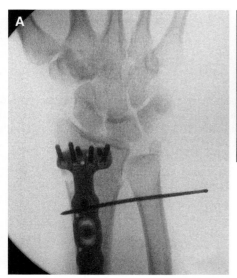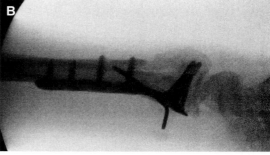

Fig. 7. Status post open reduction internal fixation of the distal radius fracture and distal radioulnar joint pinning. (*A*) Posteroanterior wrist radiograph. (*B*) Lateral wrist radiograph.

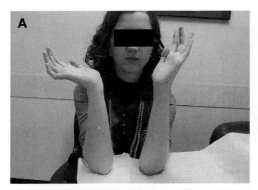

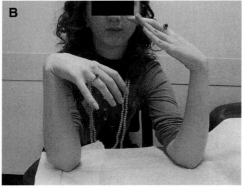

Fig. 8. Clinical range of motion 9 months postoperatively despite aggressive physiotherapy. Painful, restricted range of motion in extension (*A*) and flexion (*B*).

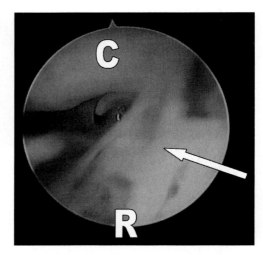

Fig. 10. Arthroscopic view from the 3-4 portal of radiocarpal adhesions (Type IA wrist arthrofibrosis). (C, carpus; R, radius; *arrow*: adhesions).

information. Examination should be performed in both the posteroanterior (PA) and lateral planes with the wrist moving in flexion-extension and radial and ulnar deviation. Lack of combined motion through both the radiocarpal and midcarpal joints is suggestive, although not necessarily diagnostic, of arthrofibrosis, as the proximal carpal row is being "fixed" and restrained. The examiner will note motion through the midcarpal joint only

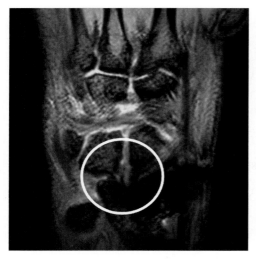

Fig. 9. MRI appearance of arthrofibrosis. Fibrous bands (encircled) extend from the radius to the carpus (Type IA wrist arthrofibrosis).

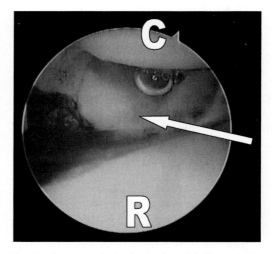

Fig. 11. Status postlysis of adhesions debridement. The radiocarpal joint has been freed of the "spot welding" effect. (C, carpus; R, radius; *arrow*: free space after lysis of adhesions debridement.)

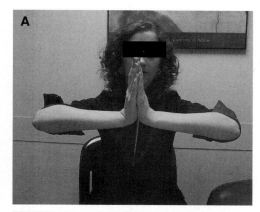

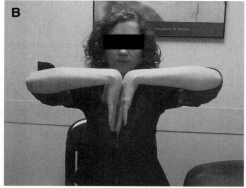

Fig. 12. After arthroscopic release, range of motion improved dramatically in both extension (*A*) and flexion (*B*).

on flexion-extension in the lateral view. This is confirmed by the absence of reciprocal motion of the proximal carpal row with radial and ulnar deviation of the PA examination.

For radiocarpal and midcarpal adhesions (Types IA and IB, respectively), the definitive diagnostic study and treatment is wrist arthroscopy. With arthrofibrosis, one notes discrete, thick, fibrous bands "spot welding" the radius to the scaphoid or lunate. These can be resected through conventional 3-4, 4-5, 6R, 6U, MCR, and MCU portals. However, capsular thickening, analogous to adhesive capsulitis of the shoulder, may also be present. If so, resection of the affected tissue done in an open manner as advocated by Watson and Weinzweig [14], or done arthroscopically as advocated by Verhellen and Bain [44], may be performed. If performed arthroscopically, the surgeon must be prepared to access the wrist by means of a palmar radial portal to adequately visualize and resect the dorsal capsule. The open

technique may permit preservation of the important palmar ligaments, but does not permit resection of intraarticular adhesions. Arthroscopic release is excellent for intraarticular adhesions. Therefore, in select cases, a combined approach may be helpful. Midcarpal arthroscopy should also routinely be included in the procedure.

Persistent limitation of motion after wrist trauma may be treatable. Most patients will respond to aggressive therapy, splinting, and cortisone injections, and improvement may continue for 12 to 18 months after injury. However, for the recidivistic wrist, a nihilistic approach is not, necessarily, warranted in a properly motivated patient with demonstrable arthrofibrosis. Aggressive debridement of arthrofibrotic tissue and, if necessary, thickened, scarred capsule, may be beneficial.

References

[1] Sprague NF III, O'Connor RL, Fox JM. Arthroscopic treatment of postoperative knee arthrofibrosis. Clin Orthop Relat Res 1982;66:165–72.

[2] Hughston JC. Complications of anterior cruciate ligament surgery. Orthop Clin North Am 1985;16:237–40.

[3] Parisien JS. The role of arthroscopy in the treatment of postoperative fibroarthrosis of the knee joint. Clin Orthop Relat Res 1988;229:185–92.

[4] Shelbourne KD, Wilckens JH, Mollabashy A, et al. Arthrofibrosis in acute anterior cruciate ligament reconstruction: The effect of timing of reconstruction and rehabilitation. Am J Sports Med 1991;19:332–6.

[5] Strohmeyer KC, Wilckens JH, Burkhalter W Jr, et al. Destructive posttraumatic subtalar synovitis. Am J Orthop 2002;31:349–52.

[6] El Rassi G, Riddle EC, Kumar SJ. Arthrofibrosis involving the middle facet of the talocalcaneal joint in children and adolescents. J Bone Joint Surg 2005;87A:2227–31.

[7] Diwan DB, Murrell GA. An evaluation of the effects of the extent of capsular release and of postoperative therapy on the temporal outcomes of adhesive capsulitis. Arthroscopy 2005;21(9):1105–13.

[8] Grey RG. The natural history of "idiopathic" frozen shoulder. J Bone Joint Surg 1978;60A:564.

[9] Nicholson GP. Arthroscopic capsular release for stiff shoulders: effect of etiology on outcomes. Arthroscopy 2003;19:40–9.

[10] Warner JJ, Allen AA, Marks PH, et al. Arthroscopic release of post-operative capsular contracture of the shoulder. J Bone Joint Surg 1997;79A:1151–8.

[11] Jones GS, Savoie FH 3rd. Arthroscopic capsular release of flexion contractures (arthrofibrosis) of the elbow. Arthroscopy 1993;9:277–83.

[12] Philips BB, Strasburger S. Arthroscopic treatment of arthrofibrosis of the elbow joint. Arthroscopy 1998; 14:38–44.

[13] Shelbourne KD, Patel DV, Martini DJ. Classification and management of arthrofibrosis of the knee after anterior cruciate ligament reconstruction. Am J Sports Med 1996;24:857–62.

[14] Watson HK, Weinzweig J. Stiff joints. In: Green DP, Hotchkiss RN, Pederson WC, editors. Green's operative hand surgery. 4th edition. New York: Churchill Livingston; 1999. p. 559.

[15] Bain GI, Richards RS, Roth JH. Wrist arthroscopy. In: Lichtman DM, Alexander AH, editors. The wrist and its disorders. Philadelphia (PA): WB Saunders; 1997. p. 151–68.

[16] Yu HL, Chase RA, Strauch B. Terminology for functions and movements of the hand. In: Yu HL, Chase RA, Strauch B, editors. Atlas of hand anatomy and clinical implications. St Louis (MO): Mosby; 2004. p. 16–42.

[17] Palmer AK, Werner FW, Murphy D, et al. Functional wrist motion: a biomechanical study. J Hand Surg 1985;10A:39–46.

[18] Morrey BF, Askew LJ, Chao EY. A biomechanical study of normal functional elbow motion. J Bone Joint Surg 1981;63A:872–7.

[19] Ryu JY, Cooney WP 3rd, Askew LJ, et al. Functional ranges of motion of the wrist joint. J Hand Surg 1991;16A:409–19.

[20] Adams DA, Grosland NM, Murphy DM, et al. Impact of impaired wrist motion on hand and upper-extremity performance. J Hand Surg 2003;28A: 898–903.

[21] Cooney WP. Contractures of the elbow. In: Morrey BF, editor. The elbow and its disorders. Philadelphia (PA): WB Saunders; 1993. p. 464–75.

[22] Bosch U. Arthrofibrosis. Orthopade 2002;31: 785–90.

[23] Bosch U, Zeichen J, Lobenhoffer P, et al. Etiology of arthrofibrosis. Arthroscopie 1999;12:215–21.

[24] Bosch U, Zeichen J, Lobenhoffer P, et al. Arthrofibrosis—a chronic inflammatory process? Arthroscopie 1999;12:117–20.

[25] Paulos LE, Rosenberg TD, Drawbert J, et al. Infrapatellar contracture syndrome: an unrecognized cause of knee stiffness with patella entrapment and patella infera. Am J Sport Med 1987;15: 331–41.

[26] Shelbourne KD, Patel DV. Treatment of limited motion after anterior cruciate ligament reconstruction. Knee Surg Sports Traumatol Arthrosc 1999;7: 85–92.

[27] Zeichen J, van Griensven M, Albers I, et al. Immunohistochemical localization of collagen VI in arthrofibrosis. Arch Orthop Trauma Surg 1999; 119:315–8.

[28] Bosch U, Zeichen J, Skutek M, et al. Arthrofibrosis is the result of a T cell mediated immune response. Knee Surg Sports Traumatol Arthrosc 2001;9:282–9.

[29] Skutek M, Elsner HA, Slateva K, et al. Screening for arthrofibrosis after anterior cruciate ligament reconstruction: analysis of association with human leukocyte antigen. Arthroscopy 2004;20:469–73.

[30] Border WA, Noble N. Transforming growth factor b in tissue fibrosis. N Engl J Med 1994;331:1286–92.

[31] Border WA, Ruoslahti E. Transforming growth factor b in disease: the dark side of tissue repair. J Clin Invest 1992;90:1–7.

[32] Unterhauser FN, Bosch U, Zeichen J, Weiler A. Alfa-smooth muscle actin containing contractile fibroblastic cells in human knee arthrofibrosis tissue. Arch Orthop Trauma Surg 2004;124:585–91.

[33] Kaplan FTD. Stiffness and joint contracture. In: Friedman SL, editor. Complications in orthopaedics—distal radius fractures. Rosemont (IL): American Academy of Orthopaedic Surgeons; 2005. p. 45–54.

[34] Prosser R. Splinting in the management of proximal interphalangeal joint flexion contracture. J Hand Ther 1996;9:378–86.

[35] Bonutti PM, Windau JE, Ables BA, et al. Static progressive stretch to reestablish elbow range of motion. Clin Orthop Relat Res 1994;303:128–34.

[36] Warner JJ, Allen A, Marks PH, et al. Arthroscopic release for chronic, refractory adhesive capsulitis of the shoulder. J Bone Joint Surg 1996;78A:1808–16.

[37] Richmond JC, al Assal M. Arthroscopic management of arthrofibrosis of the knee, including infrapatellar contraction syndrome. Arthroscopy 1991;7: 144–7.

[38] Lapner PC, Leith JM, Regan WD. Arthroscopic debridement of the elbow for arthrofibrosis resulting from nondisplaced fracture of the radial head. Arthroscopy 2005;21:1492.

[39] Zanotti RM, Kuhn JE. Arthroscopic capsular release for the stiff shoulder. Description of technique and anatomic considerations. Am J Sports Med 1997;25:294–8.

[40] Hattori T, Hirata H, Nakao E, et al. Arthroscopic mobilization for post-traumatic contracture of the wrist. American Society for Surgery of the Hand Annual Meeting Abstracts, Washington, DC, Sept. 7–9, 2006.

[41] Slutsky DJ. Wrist arthroscopy through a volar radial portal. Arthroscopy 2002;18:624–30.

[42] Kleinman WB, Graham TJ. The distal radioulnar joint capsule: clinical anatomy and role in posttraumatic limitation of forearm rotation. J Hand Surg 1998;23A:588–99.

[43] Kleinman WB. DRUJ contracture release. Tech Hand Up Extrem Surg 1999;3:13–22.

[44] Verhellen R, Bain GI. Arthroscopic capsular release for contracture of the wrist: a new technique. Arthroscopy 2000;16:106–10.

[45] Viegas SF, Patterson RM, Ward K. Extrinsic wrist ligaments in the pathomechanics of ulnar translation instability. J Hand Surg 1995;20A:312–8.

Index

Note: Page numbers of article titles are in **boldface** type.

United States Postal Service
Statement of Ownership, Management, and Circulation

1. Publication Title	2. Publication Number		3. Filing Date
Hand Clinics	0 0 0 - 7 0 9		9/15/06

4. Issue Frequency	5. Number of Issues Published Annually	6. Annual Subscription Price
Feb, May, Aug, Nov	4	$215.00

7. Complete Mailing Address of Known Office of Publication *(Not printer) (Street, city, county, state, and ZIP+4)*

Elsevier Inc.
360 Park Avenue South
New York, NY 10010-1710

Contact Person
Sam Carmichael
Telephone
(215) 239-3681

8. Complete Mailing Address of Headquarters or General Business Office of Publisher *(Not printer)*

Elsevier Inc., 360 Park Avenue South, New York, NY 10010-1710

9. Full Names and Complete Mailing Addresses of Publisher, Editor, and Managing Editor *(Do not leave blank)*

Publisher *(Name and complete mailing address)*

John Schrefer, Elsevier Inc., 1600 John F. Kennedy Blvd., Suite 1800, Philadelphia, PA 19103-2899

Editor *(Name and complete mailing address)*

Debora Dellapena, Elsevier Inc., 1600 John F. Kennedy Blvd., Suite 1800, Philadelphia, PA 19103-2899

Managing Editor *(Name and complete mailing address)*

Catherine Bewick, Elsevier Inc., 1600 John F. Kennedy Blvd., Suite 1800, Philadelphia, PA 19103-2899

10. Owner *(Do not leave blank. If the publication is owned by a corporation, give the name and address of the corporation immediately followed by the names and addresses of all stockholders owning or holding 1 percent or more of the total amount of stock. If not owned by a corporation, give the names and addresses of the individual owners. If owned by a partnership or other unincorporated firm, give its name and address as well as those of each individual owner. If the publication is published by a nonprofit organization, give its name and address.)*

Full Name	Complete Mailing Address
Wholly owned subsidiary of	4520 East-West Highway
Reed/Elsevier Inc, US holdings	Bethesda, MD 20814

11. Known Bondholders, Mortgagees, and Other Security Holders Owning or Holding 1 Percent or More of Total Amount of Bonds, Mortgages, or Other Securities. If none, check box ▶ None

Full Name	Complete Mailing Address
N/A	

12. Tax Status *(For completion by nonprofit organizations authorized to mail at nonprofit rates) (Check one)*
The purpose, function, and nonprofit status of this organization and the exempt status for federal income tax purposes:
☐ Has Not Changed During Preceding 12 Months
☐ Has Changed During Preceding 12 Months *(Publisher must submit explanation of change with this statement)*

(See Instructions on Reverse)

PS Form **3526**, October 1999

---

13. Publication Title	14. Issue Date for Circulation Data Below
Hand Clinics	August, 2006

15.	Extent and Nature of Circulation		Average No. Copies Each Issue During Preceding 12 Months	No. Copies of Single Issue Published Nearest to Filing Date
a.	Total Number of Copies *(Net press run)*		2,700	2,600
b. Paid and/or Requested Circulation	(1)	Paid/Requested Outside-County Mail Subscriptions Stated on Form 3541. *(Include advertiser's proof and exchange copies)*	1,476	1,390
	(2)	Paid In-County Subscriptions Stated on Form 3541 *(Include advertiser's proof and exchange copies)*		
	(3)	Sales Through Dealers and Carriers, Street Vendors, Counter Sales, and Other Non-USPS Paid Distribution	467	490
	(4)	Other Classes Mailed Through the USPS		
c.	Total Paid and/or Requested Circulation *[Sum of 15b. (1), (2), (3), and (4)]* ▶		1,943	1,880
d. Free Distribution by Mail *(Samples, complimentary, and other free)*	(1)	Outside-County as Stated on Form 3541	115	114
	(2)	In-County as Stated on Form 3541		
	(3)	Other Classes Mailed Through the USPS		
e.	Free Distribution Outside the Mail *(Carriers or other means)*			
f.	Total Free Distribution *(Sum of 15d. and 15e.)* ▶		115	114
g.	Total Distribution *(Sum of 15c. and 15f)* ▶		2,058	1,994
h.	Copies not Distributed		642	606
i.	Total *(Sum of 15g. and h.)* ▶		2,700	2,600
j.	Percent Paid and/or Requested Circulation *(15c. divided by 15g. times 100)*		94.41%	94.28%

16. Publication of Statement of Ownership
☐ Publication required. Will be printed in the November 2006 issue of this publication.
☐ Publication not required

17. Signature and Title of Editor, Publisher, Business Manager, or Owner

[signature] John Fanucci – Executive Director of Subscription Services

Date 9/15/06

I certify that all information furnished on this form is true and complete. I understand that anyone who furnishes false or misleading information on this form or who omits material or information requested on the form may be subject to criminal sanctions (including fines and imprisonment) and/or civil sanctions (including civil penalties).

Instructions to Publishers

1. Complete and file one copy of this form with your postmaster annually on or before October 1. Keep a copy of the completed form for your records.
2. In cases where the stockholder or security holder is a trustee, include in items 10 and 11 the name of the person or corporation for whom the trustee is acting. Also include the names and addresses of individuals who are stockholders who own or hold 1 percent or more of the total amount of bonds, mortgages, or other securities of the publishing corporation. In item 11, if none, check the box. Use blank sheets if more space is required.
3. Be sure to furnish all circulation information called for in item 15. Free circulation must be shown in items 15d, e, and f.
4. Item 15h, Copies not Distributed, must include (1) newsstand copies originally stated on Form 3541, and returned to the publisher, (2) estimated returns from news agents, and (3), copies for office use, leftovers, spoiled, and all other copies not distributed.
5. If the publication had Periodicals authorization as a general or requester publication, this Statement of Ownership, Management, and Circulation must be published; it must be printed in any issue in October or, if the publication is not published during October, the first issue printed after October.
6. In item 16, indicate the date of the issue in which this Statement of Ownership will be published.
7. Item 17 must be signed.

Failure to file or publish a statement of ownership may lead to suspension of Periodicals authorization.

PS Form **3526**, October 1999 *(Reverse)*

Moving?

Make sure your subscription moves with you!

To notify us of your new address, find your **Clinics Account Number** (located on your mailing label above your name), and contact customer service at:

E-mail: elspcs@elsevier.com

800-654-2452 (subscribers in the U.S. & Canada)
407-345-4000 (subscribers outside of the U.S. & Canada)

Fax number: 407-363-9661

Elsevier Periodicals Customer Service
6277 Sea Harbor Drive
Orlando, FL 32887-4800

*To ensure uninterrupted delivery of your subscription, please notify us at least 4 weeks in advance of move.